Modulation Of Sialidases In Pancreatic Cancer

Shalini Nath

Index

Chapter VI...

CHAPTER I

Introduction

1.0 Cancer

Uncontrolled proliferating cells give rise to tumors which is a mass of cell present in a tissue. Growth of tumor mainly interacts and communicates with various systems (eg. digestive, nervous, and circulatory systems) in human body, thus giving them signal to release hormones and chemicals to enhance the growth of tumor[1].

Tumors are of two types, Benign that stays in one spot with limited growth and malignant, the dangerous type. Cancerous cells escapes from the solid tumor mass and travel within blood or lymphatic systems to invade in healthy tissue. There these cancerous cells manage to proliferate and grow with the help of newly formed blood vessel by the process called angiogenesis.

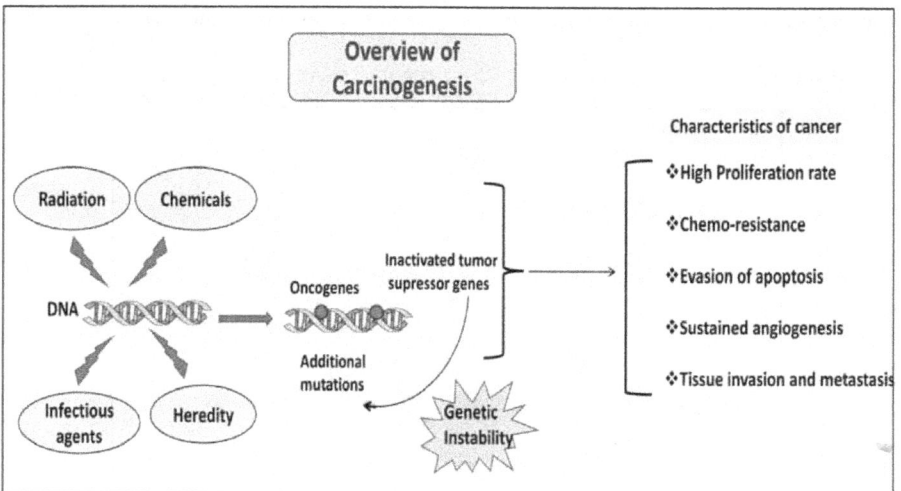

Figure 1.1 Overview of carcinogenesis. Image downloaded from https://www.slideshare.net/meducationdotnet/principles-of-oncology.

The malignant tumor that spreads and invade in another healthy tissue within a body give rise to another tumor, by the process called metastatsis[2,3]. Metastasized tumor are very hard to treat even after various cancer treatments like chemotherapy, radiation, and/or surgery due to their chemo resistance and their diffuse localization in different organs which causes relapse of the cancer (Fig. 1.1). Among the 100 types of cancer that is reported till date[3] my main focus is on pancreatic ductal adenocarcinoma (PDAC) which I will provide in depth study.

1.1 Pancreas

Pancreas is part of digestive as well as endocrine system. It is a heterocrine gland. It secretes hormones like insulin, glucagon, somatostatin, and pancreatic polypeptide as a endocrine gland.

It secretes many digestive enzymes which catabolises carbohydrates, proteins and fats in stomach. It also secretes bicarbonate containing pancreatic juice into the duodenum to neutralizes acid[4-6]. Thus pancreas serves as also a exocrine gland.

Pancreas is located in the upper left part of abdomen. Pancreas can be divided into head, neck, body, and tail measuring 12–15 centimetres in adults (Fig. 1.2).

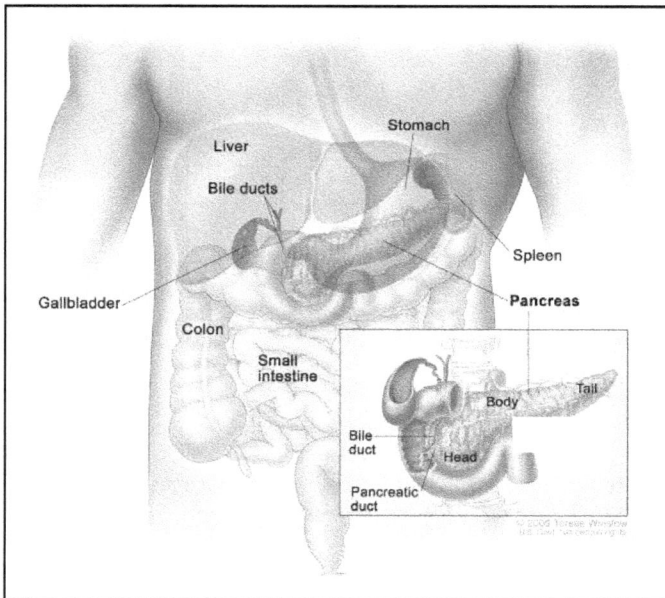

Figure 1.2 Anatomy of pancreas. Image downloaded from https://www.ohsu.edu/knight-cancer-institute/understanding-pancreatic-cancer

1.2 Pancreatic cancer

Pancreatic cancer is the 7th highest cause of death by cancer in the world (Fig. 1.3)[7,8]. Due to difficulty in early diagnosis and its rapid growth it shows very poor survival rates of five years. Only 2%-9% patients survive[9,10.] It generally occurs by mutation in the pancreatic cells and generally metastasized to nearby organs through its connecting blood vessels (Fig. 1.4). There are no early stage specific symptoms detected in this deadly disease, even when patient felt the symptoms it had already been metastasized and spread in several organs within body[11-14].

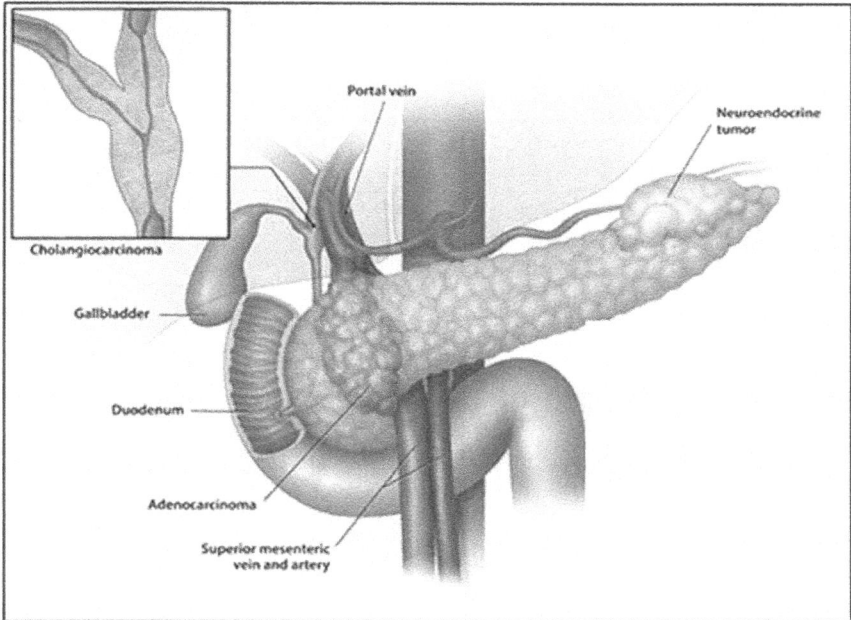

Figure 1.3 Different types of pancreatic cancer. Image downloaded from https://columbiasurgery.org/conditions-and-treatments/pancreatic-cancer

1.2A Type and characteristics of pancreatic cancer

95% pancreatic tumors are mostly exocrine, whereas only 5% of pancreatic tumors are endocrine[15,16].

- Pancreatic ductal adenocarcinoma (PDAC), is an exocrine tumour which mainly occurs in exocrine cells that secrete digestive enzymes.

- Neuroendocrine tumours in pancreas known as PNETs or pancNETS occur in endocrine cells that produce hormones like insulin.

Normal Duct   PanIN1A   PanIN2   PanIN3   Adenocarcinoma

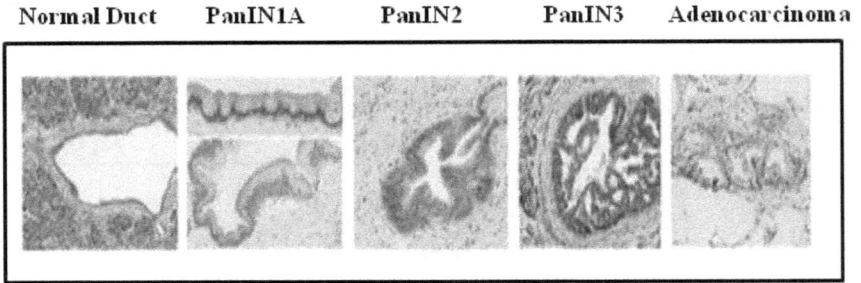

Figure 1.4 Histological images of pancreatic intraepithelial neoplasias (PanINs) representing different stages of pancreatic adenocarcinoma. The image have been downloaded from https://www.nature.com/articles/nrc949/figures/2

1.2B Risk factors associated with pancreatic cancer

The risk factors that are associated with PDAC are mostly with genetic syndromes[17]. Most common mutation that occurs in PDAC is hyperactivated KRAS gene which helps in the uncontrolled proliferation of cells. This mutation also helps in metastasis. Along with KRAS mutation, inactivating mutations of CDKN2A, p53, and SMAD family member 4 (SMAD4) tumor suppressors are detected in high grade tumors. Germline mutations in BRCA2 can also cause pancreatic cancer, along with breast, ovarian cancer[17,18]. Several environmental factors also affect the development of pancreatic cancer for eg. smoking, long-standing diabetes mellitus, nonhereditary and chronic pancreatitis[18].

1.2C Age and gender

The risk of developing pancreatic cancer increases with age[19]. It generally develops between the age group of 60-80 years. It is more common in men because men are more likely to smoke tobacco (Fig. 1.5)

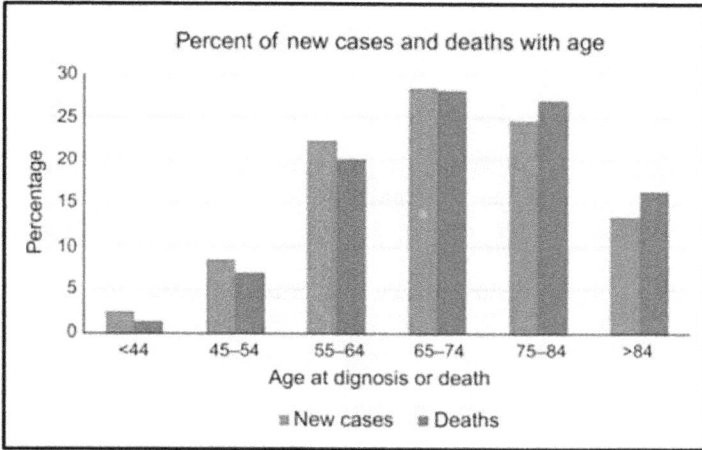

Figure 1.5 Percentage of new cases and death by pancreatic cancer among various age groups. Image downloaded from https://www.sciencedirect.com/ science/article/pii/B9780128176610000020

1.2D Race

Studies show that pancreatic cancer prevalence is mostly in North-America. It is more common in African-american population than in white population[20] (Fig. 1.6).

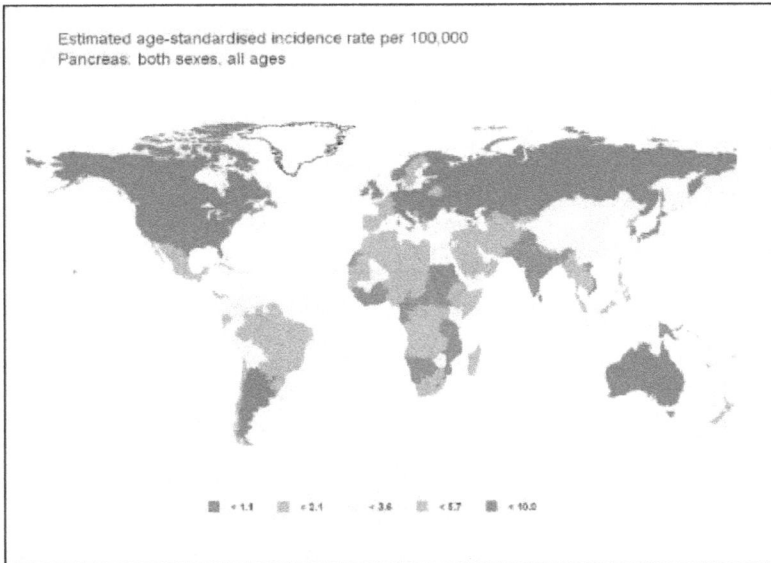

Figure 1.6 Epidemiology of pancreatic cancer. Image downloaded from *Gastroenterol Hepatol Bed Bench. 2017 Fall;10(4):245-257.*

1.3 Cancer stem cells in pancreatic cancer

Cancer stem cells (CSCs) are the main culprit in resistance to anticancer treatment, metastasis and relapse of cancer including PDAC. These are mainly immortal in nature which have properties like self-renew, can give rise to several different progenitor cells and form malignant tumors[21,22]. Higher expression levels of anti-apoptotic proteins, ABC transporters, and multidrug resistance genes are found in CSCs. Pancreatic cancer stem cells (pCSCs) was first described in the year 2007. These pCSCs mainly responsible for relapse, chemo-resistance and tumor growth/progression. The markers needed for identifying pCSCs are commonly CD133 and CD44. The main signalling pathways that have been implemented in maintenance of stemness are Hedgehog (Hh), Wnt/β-catenin and Notch. Other several pathway that enhance the robustness of pCSCs are mammalian target of rapamycin (mTOR), Bmi-1, NODAL/ACTIVIN, NF-κB and PTEN pathways. CSCs mainly involved in chemi-resistance by the processes of efflux of drugs, and mutations of several oncogenes and tumor suppressor genes which lead to inactivation of several drug targets. Also in CSCs up-regulation of aldehyde dehydrogenase and proteasome, reduction of the human equilibrative nucleoside transporters (ENTs) and human concentrative nucleoside transporters (CNTs) were found which play major role in chemo-resistance. Therefore, further research is very much needed for the development of new drugs to target pCSCs[23-25].

1.4 Therapies used in pancreatic cancer

As for prognostic indicator and to decide therapy, tumor grading is done in pancreatic cancer post resection of tumor[26]. Pancreatic cancer is currently staged on the basis of 6th edition of the *AJCC Cancer Staging Manual,* which was published in 2002 (Table 1.1).

Tumor node metastasis (TNM) classification of pancreatic cancer	
Primary tumor (T stage)	
TX	Primary tumor cannot be evaluated
T0	No confirmation of primary tumor
Tis	Carcinoma in situ
T1	Tumor limited to pancreas with less than 2cm diameter
T2	Tumor limited to pancreas with greater than 2cm diameter
T3	Tumor enlarged beyond pancreas
T4	Tumor enlarged beyond pancreas which mainly involves superior mesenteric artery (no resection possibility)
N stage (regional lymph nodes)	
NX	Regional nodes can not be found
N0	Absence of regional lymph node metastasis
N1	Presence of regional lymph node metastasis
M stage (distant sites)	
M0	Distant metastasis not found
M1	Distant metastasis is found

Table 1.1 TNM staging system of pancreatic cancer proposed by American Joint Committee on Cancer (AJCC) 6th edition.

In most of the cases in early stage of pancreatic cancer shows no sign at all. However, five symptoms mainly occur during progression of pancreatic cancer like back/shoulder pain, dysphagia, lethargy, weight loss[27]. Therapies that have been used in pancreatic cancer (Fig. 1.7) are given below.

- **Surgical resection** till now is the only mode of treatment in pancreatic cancer which increases the chance of survival of patients. *Pancreatoduodenectomy* is removal of tumor from head of pancreas, whereas removal of tumors from pancreatic body and tail known as *pancreatectomy*.

- **Radiation therapy** with the help of X-ray and protons cancer cells are destroyed.

- **Chemotherapy** the drug Gemcitabine is mainly given orally or directly administered in vein by injection, when the cancer has been metastasized.

- **Combination therapy** combinations of all these therapies also give better control of this disease. Hence, effective drugs are very much needed to combat this deadly disease.

- **Neoadjuvant chemotherapy** is when chemotherapy is given before resection of tumor.

- **Adjuvant chemotherapy** here chemotherapy and radiation, or chemotherapy and surgery are used together.

Identifications of new drug targets are required for target specific therapies in pancreatic cancer. Development of new drugs is very much needed for the treatment of pancreatic cancer as there are only few drugs are present[28-32].

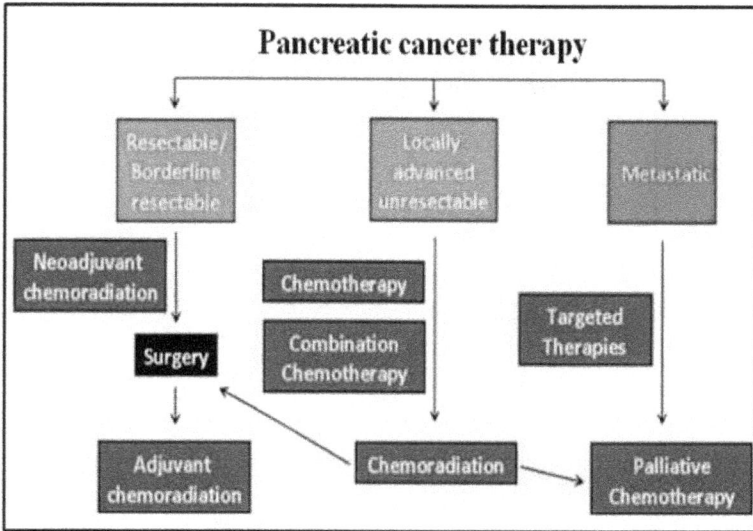

Figure 1.7 Therapies used in pancreatic cancer. This image is downloaded from www.sciencedirect.com/science/article/pii/B9780124081031000030

1.5 Sialylation in pancreatic cancer

The process of sialylation involves addition of sialic acids at the terminal position on oligosaccharides and carbohydrates moieties. Sialic acids are commonly known as N-acetylneuraminic acid (Neu5Ac or NANA) with a nine-carbon backbone[33-36].

Up-regulation of α2,3- and α2,6-linkage specific sialylation is found in pancreatic cancer which helps in the progression of cancer[37,38] (Fig. 1.8). Level of sialylation is modulated by sialyltransferases and sialidases[39-41].

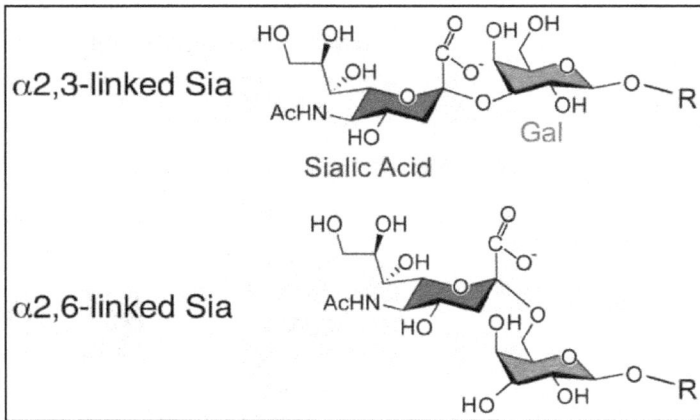

Figure 1.8 The structure of sialic acid with different linkages. Image downloaded from Int J Mol Sci. 2017 Jul; 18(7): 1541.

1.6 Biosynthesis of sialic acids

Sialic acid biosynthesis takes place in cytoplasm (Fig. 1.9). Glucose breaks down and forms UDP-GlcNAc which is a main substrate for the biosynthesis of sialic acids. UDP-GlcNAc 2-epimerase then converts UDP-GlcNAc into ManNAc. Then ManNAc kinase helps in the phosphorylation of ManNAc. CMP-sialic acid synthease which activates sialic acids present is the nucleus. This CMP-sialic acid synthease donates sialic acids to glycans on glycoproteins or glycolipids in the Golgi[42]. It also acts as an inhibitor of the UDP-GlcNAc 2-epimerase enzyme by binding to its allosteric site by feedback loop which is the rate limiting step[43,44].

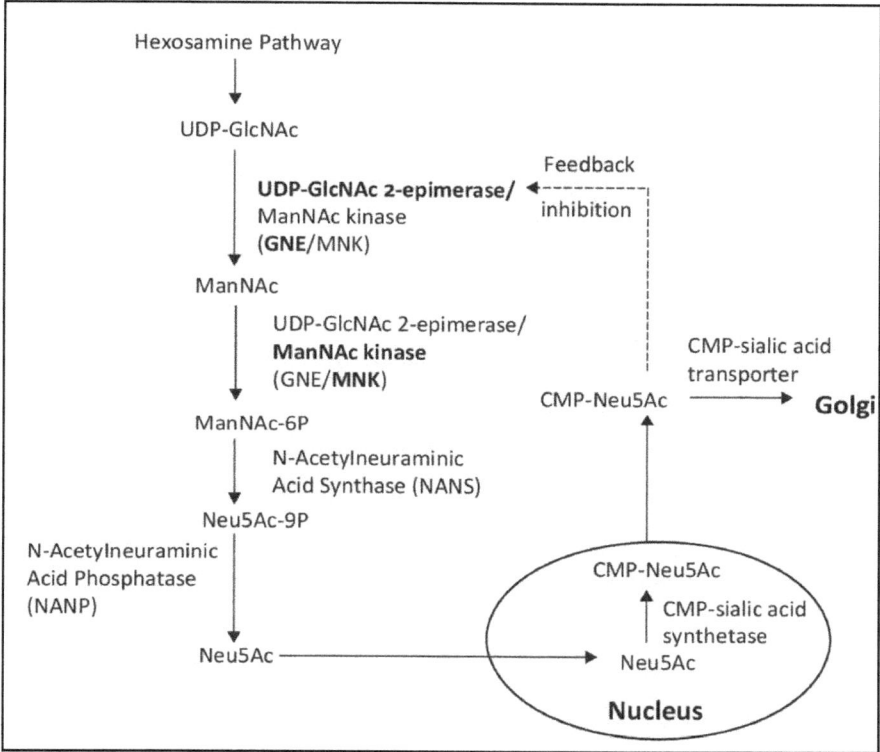

Figure 1.9 Biosynthesis of sialic acids. Image downloaded from Methods Mol Biol. 2017; 1603:25-44.

1.7 Location of sialylation process

Sialylation is essential for many different cellular processes like development, regulation of immune responses, cell differentiation, cancer progression[45-47]. Generally sialic acids are found on the terminal position of N- and O-linked glycoproteins and glycolipids (Fig. 1.10).

In case of N-linked glycan, N-acetyl glucosamine (GlcNAc) is attached to the amide nitrogen of an asparagine, whereas in O-linked the glycan, N-acetyl galactosamine (GalNAc) is attached to oxygen of a serine or threonine side chain. C-3 or C-6 positions of galactose residues or to the C-6 position of *N*-acetylgalactosamine residues are the most common linkages [47-49].

Sialylation is a post translational modification which mainly occurs in Golgi complex (Fig. 1.11). The modification of sialylation is maintained by retrograde vesicle trafficking within Golgi cisternae. Different types of linkage specific sialyltransferases (STs) catalyze the reaction to transfer sialic acids from CMP-sialic acids in Golgi cisternaes. The localization of STs, which are type II membrane proteins within Golgi are dependent upon complex signals[50-53].

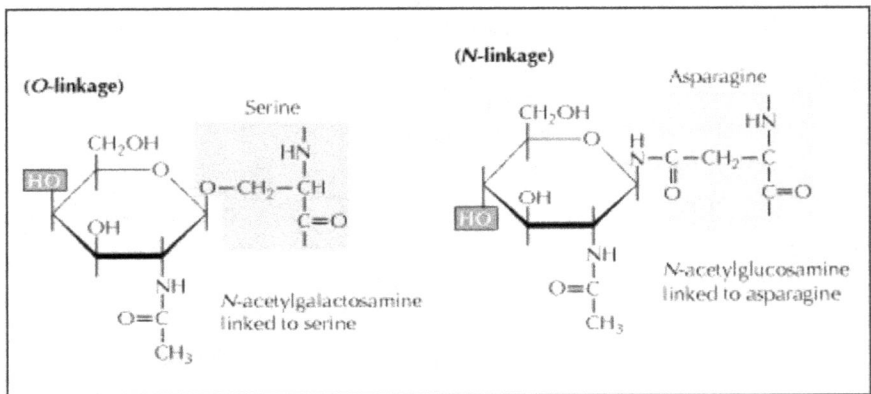

Figure 1.10 O- and N- linked glycosylation. Image downloaded from http://www.premierbiosoft.com/glycan/glossary/glycosylation.html

1.8 Sialic acid modulatory enzymes

The balance of sialylation within eukaryotic cells are maintained by mainly two enzymes sialyltransferases and sialidases (Fig. 1.11). STs mainly add sialic acids to the glycoproteins, glycolipids and oligosaccharides[54,55]. There are probably more than twenty different types of sialyltransferases are present in eukaryotes having different substrate specificity [56-61].

Sialidases catalyze the removal of α2,3- and α2,6- glycosidic linkages from sialylated glycoproteins, glycolipids and oligosaccharides[62]. There are four different types of sialidase in eukaryotes having different location in the cell and substrate specificity[63-66].

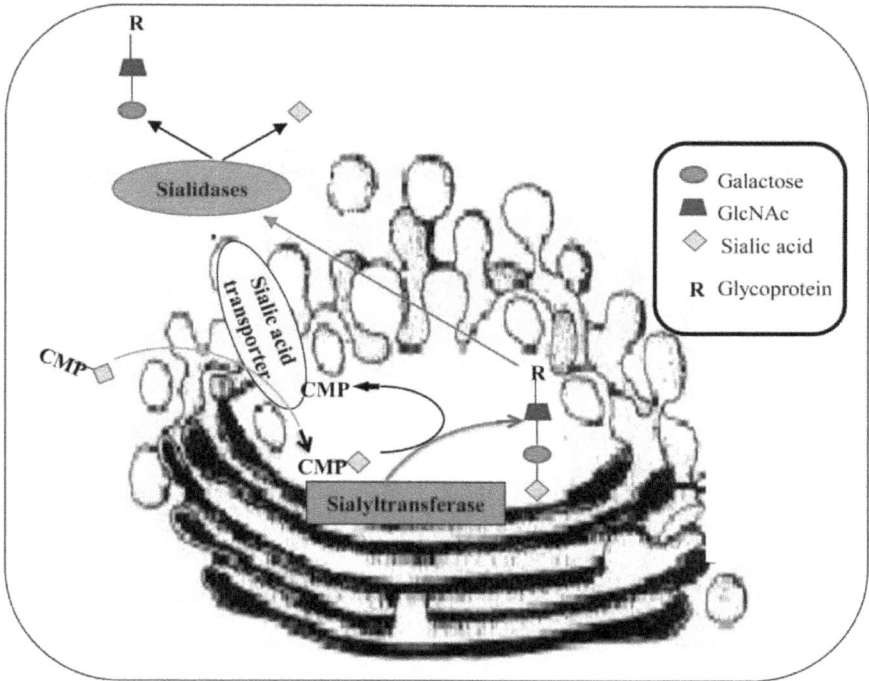

Figure 1.11 Schematic representation of regulation and location of the process sialylation

1.8A Sialyltransferases

Sialyltransferases play an important role during the maintenance of sialylation within cells. Imbalance of sialylation generally associated with different disease conditions like during carcinogenesis[67-68]. It has been observed that during cancer the level of sialylation have been up-regulated and further studies provide information that during cancer one of the reason for the up-regulation of sialylation is the enhanced expression of sialyltransferases[69-75]. Several different types of sialyltransferases have been involved in various cancers as mentioned in Table

1.2.

Sialyltransferases	Types of cancers in which the altered expression observed	References
ST3Gal I	Breast, bladder, colon	76-78
ST3Gal II	Prostate, colon	78,79
ST3Gal III	Stomach, pancreas, extrahepatic bile duct, cervix	80-83
ST3Gal IV	Renal cell, stomach	84,85
ST3Gal V	Pediatric leukemia	86
ST6Gal I	Colon, breast, cervix, choriocarcinomas, acute myeloid leukemias, liver, brain	87-96
ST6GalNAc I	Stomach, pancreas, colon, ovary, breast	97-100
ST6GalNAc II	Colon	98-101
ST6GalNAc V	Colon, breast	102,103
ST6GalNAc VI	Colon	104
ST8Sia I	Breast cancer, pediatric acute leukemia	105
ST8Sia II	Liver	93
ST8Sia III	Glioblastoma	106

Table 1.2 Involvement of sialyltransferases in human cancers (Molecules. 2015 20: 7509–7527)

1.8B Sialidases

In mammalian system, there are four different types of sialidases or neuraminidases known till date designated as Neu1, Neu2, Neu3, Neu4. They are mainly coded by different genes. The characteristic features of these four sialidase have been mentioned in Table 1.3. Each sialidases play different role during carcinogenesis due to their differential expression which causes enhanced sialylation[107].

Sub-cellular	**Neu1**	**Neu2**	**Neu3**	**Neu4**
localization	lysosomes	cytosol	Plasma membrane	Lumen of Lysosomes, mitochondria, ER
Substrates	Oligosaccharides glycopeptides	Oligosaccharide glycopeptides, gangliosides	gangliosides	Oligosaccharides, glycopeptides, gangliosides
Amino acids in human sialidases	409	380	428	496
Linkage specificity	α2,3	α2,3 and α2,6	α2,3	α2,3 and α2,6
Optimal pH (in vitro)	4.4-4.6	5.6-6.5	4.6-4.8	3.2-4.5

Table 1.3 Characteristics of mammalian sialidases

Modulation of sialylation in cancer cells leads to control the effectiveness of anticancer drugs and chemotherapy. The resistance of cancer chemotherapy which is sialidase-mediated leads to up-regulation of several multidrug resistance genes like ABCC1, ABCC3, ABCC5 and ABCB1 system in cancer[108-110].

I. Neu1 in cancer

Neu1 is a lysosomal sialidase which forms a complex with carboxypeptidase A and β-galactosidase, the dissociation of this complex leads to inactivation of Neu[111]. C-terminal motif that present in Neu1 helps for its localization and transport to lysosomes[112]. NEU1 desialylates PDGF and IGF-1 receptors which leads to reduce the growth of aortic smooth muscle cells and fibroblasts[113]. It has been reported that Neu1 along with matrix metalloproteinase-9 in plasma membrane helps in the activation of NGF-induced Trk tyrosine kinase receptor and up-regulation of cell signalling processes suggesting Neu1 can move to plasma membrane and desialylate several surface molecule important for cellular signalling[114]. Also, another few studies suggest that in different conditions this sialidase often localizes in plasma membrane as well as in lysosomes. Hence, the location of Neu1 within cell varies.

Cancers like melanoma and colon adenocarcinoma have low expression of Neu1. In melanoma low expression of Neu1 causes higher metastasis at lung, also in colon adenocarcinoma showed similar trend suggesting Neu1 has a inverse relationship with metastatic potential of cancer cells In these cancers, overexpression of Neu1 causes suppression of metastasis and tumor progression by reduction of anchorage-independent growth which resulted in enhanced apoptosis[115,116].

However, interestingly, in different cancer like hepatocellular carcinoma, Neu1 is identified as oncogene due to its upregulated expression in both mRNA and protein levels which increases cell proliferation and migration[117]. Also, up-regulation of Neu1 is found in pancreatic cancer which increases cancer growth by desialylating α2,3-linked sialic acids on EGFR thus helping in its smooth dimerization and constant its activation in plasma membrane, suppression of this sialidase by its inhibitor tamiflu decrease cancer progression[118].

II. Neu2 in cancer

Neu2 is a cytosolic sialidase and it is the first sialidase which have a crystal structure captured by x-ray (Fig. 1.12). Neu2 structure has canonical six-blade β-propeller, the active site resides in a shallow crevice. When inhibitor of sialidase bind to the catalytic site of Neu2 it is surrounded by ten amino acids. Among mammalian sialidases tyrosine residue is conserved which increases the enzymatic reaction in transition state[119].

Neu2 expression is very high in muscle and neuronal and prostate cells which help in differentiation of these cells[120,121]. In myoblast cell line in the presence of Neu2, the proliferation of myogenic cells as well as myotube formation has been increased severely suggesting the effective role of Neu2 in muscle cell growth and differentiation[121]. Further studies in human rhabdomyosarcoma also shows the role of Neu2 in enhancing myogenic functions as well as myogenic differentiation[122]. In neuronal cells specifically PC12, Neu2 controls the neuronal differentiation by inducing the activation of the transcription of nerve-growth factor (NGF)[120]. However, in most of the other cancer cells the expression of Neu2 is very low or undetectable [123-125]. Studies show that over-expression of Neu2 can affect cell behaviour. Over-expression of Neu2 in melanoma cells (which have high metastatic potential) reduced the metastasis in lungs with low level of ganglioside GM3 and an increase level of lactosylceramide[126]. Also in myeloid leukemia when expression of Neu2 is up-regulated it causes apoptosis in these cells through intrinsic pathway mediated apoptosis[123]. Neu2 over-expression in these cells caused reduction of Bcr-Abl, and also reduction in Bcr-Abl-dependent Src and Lyn kinase activity probably by desialylation of several glycoproteins. Hence, these results suggest that the level of Neu2 can affect the cancer progression.

In another study, the up-regulation of Neu2 in A431 human epidermoid carcinoma cells decreased the GM3 levels but increase in cell proliferation by activation of epidermal growth factor receptors (EGFR)[127]. So, the role of Neu2 acts differently in different cancers. Therefore, further studies are needed to elucidate the role of Neu2 in carcinogenesis. Hence, I have provided in depth study about the effect of Neu2-overexpression on PDAC and pCSCs.

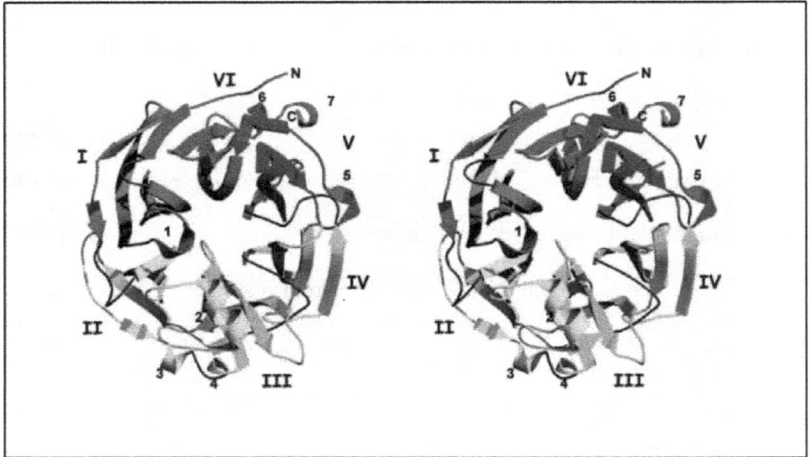

Figure 1.12 The structure of cytosolic sialidase (Neu2). A ribbon diagram. The six blades (I-VI) are differently colour coded and the loops in between them are gray coloured. Image downloaded from The Journal of Biological Chemistry 280, 469-475. http://www.jbc.org/content/280/1/469.long

III. Neu3 in cancer

Neu3 is a plasma membrane bound sialidase but sometimes it also can be found in other cellular compartments and during cellular movement in response to growth stimuli like EGF it can mobilize to membrane ruffles with Rac-1[128].

Also another report suggest that Neu3 can also be present in endosomal structures[129]. These reports suggest that the location of sialidase is not static, it can be changed in different physiological conditions within cells. The plasma membrane bound sialidase Neu3 acts in various ways in non-small cell lung cancer by controlling EGFR pathways through ERK and

Akt pathways. Hence, Neu3 can used as a biomarker for this cancer. Thus patients with high expression of Neu3 in non-small cell lung carcinoma can benefit from inhibitors of EGFR tyrosine kinase inhibitors along Akt inhibitors[130]. Neu3 was also up-regulated in head and neck squamous cancer cells which causes lymph node metastasis[131]. Interestingly expression of Neu3 is low in human fibroblast, up-regulation of this sialidase causes apoptosis[132]. Enhanced expression of Neu3 was found in prostate cancer. When Neu3 is over-expressed in LNCaP cells which has androgen-sensitive property, it induces the expression of cell proliferation specific transcription factor EGR-1 leads to cancer progression. Silencing of the Neu3 in prostate cancer by small interfering RNA caused reduction in cell growth through androgen receptor signaling pathway[133]. Also in another report knockdown of Neu3 in PC3 cells caused reduction in invasion and migration property of these cells through controlling the expressions of the matrix metalloproteinases MMP-2 and MMP-9[134]. In acute lymphoblastic leukemia the expression of Neu3 is downregulated which helps in survival of these cancer cells. Up-regulation of this sialidase in acute lymphoblastic leukemia helps to induce apoptosis[135].

IV. Neu4 in cancer

It is generally found in lumen of lysosomes and mitochondria. Neu4 expression is low in human colon cancer. During apoptosis which was induced by death ligand TRAIL this enzyme was up-regulated. Over-expression of Neu4 caused increased apoptosis and reduced migration and invasion in colon cancer by reduction of E-selectin[136]. Neu4 caused enhanced apoptosis in neuronal cells by modulating the level of gangliosided GD3 (GD3 can induce apoptosis) in neuroblastoma[137]. Interestingly, another study suggested that cell proliferation and differentiation were increased in neuroblastoma by activation of Wnt/β-catenin signaling pathway which was caused by over-expression of Neu4.

Along with this modulation of sialylation that are present on glycoproteins caused activation of several stem cell specific pluoripotent genes like MYC, NANOG, OCT-4, CD133 and NES (nestin), which caused enhanced cell proliferation and decreased differentiation[138].

In glioblastoma stem cells (GSCs), the level of Neu4 was very much up-regulated than its non-neurosphere-differentiated cells. Inhibition of Neu4 in these GSCs caused reduction in the expression of sonic hedgehog pathway molecules which known to be up-regulated in cancer stem cells. Also several stem cell specific molecules OCT4, SOX2 and NANOG, CD133 had been down-regulated after inhibition of Neu4 in GSCs. All these events lead to apoptosis in GSCs upon Neu4 inhibition[139].

1.9 Hypothesis and aims

Hence, collectively by numerous studies, it is demonstrated that abnormal sialylation is hallmark in cancer. In order to fulfill therapeutic utility by implementing new tools to control the aberrant sialylation during carcinogenesis there is an urgent need for the understanding of the molecular mechanism of the sialidases which control the degree of sialylation during cancer progression.

Expression of sialidase Neu2 is very low among most of the cancers, moreover no study have been found till date about the role of Neu2 is regulation of pancreatic cancer and pancreatic cancer stem like cells. Therefore, considering the existing evidences, the complicated interplay among several signalling molecules that have been associated with pancreatic cancer and the modulatory effect of sialylation by Neu2 on them will give the highlights of the molecular mechanism, possibly pave the way for management of pancreatic cancer and pancreatic cancer stem like cells.

References

1. Doll Richard ,Peto Richard. The Causes of Cancer: Quantitative Estimates of Avoidable Risks of Cancer in the United States Today. Journal of the National Cancer Institute 1981 June (66);1192–1308.
2. Azevedo FAC, Carvalho LRB, Grinberg LT, Farfel JM, Ferretti REL, Leite REP, et al. Equal numbers of neuronal and nonneuronal cells make the human brain an isometrically scaled-up primate brain. J Comp Neurol. 2009 Apr 10;513(5):532–41.
3. Agulhon C, Petravicz J, McMullen AB, Sweger EJ, Minton SK, Taves SR, et al. What is the role of astrocyte calcium in neurophysiology? Neuron. 2008 Sep 25;59(6):932–46.
4. Röder Pia V, Bingbing Wu,Yixian Liu, Weiping Han. Pancreatic regulation of glucose homeostasis. Exp Mol Med. 2016 Mar; 48(3): e219.
5. Chandra Rashmi, Liddle Rodger A. Modulation of Pancreatic Exocrine and Endocrine Secretion. Curr Opin Gastroenterol. 2013 Sep; 29(5): 517–522.
6. SUSSMAN KARL E. MEHLER PHILIP S., WAYNE LEITNER J. , DRAZNIN BORIS. Role of the Secretion Vesicle in the Transport of Receptors: Modulation of Somatostatin Binding to Pancreatic Islets. Endocrinology 1982 July (111):316–323.
7. lic Milena, Ilic Irena. Epidemiology of pancreatic cancer. World J Gastroenterol. 2016 Nov 28; 22(44): 9694–9705.
8. Lin Quan-Jun, Yang Feng , Jin Chen, Fu De-Liang. Current status and progress of pancreatic cancer in China. World J Gastroenterol. 2015 Jul 14; 21(26): 7988–8003.
9. Muders, M. H. et al. Expression and regulatory role of GAIP-interacting protein GIPC in pancreatic adenocarcinoma. Cancer Res. 66, 10264–10268 (2006).
10. Muders, M. H. et al. Targeting GIPC/Synectin in pancreatic cancer inhibits tumor growth. Clin. ancer 15, 4095–4103 (2009).
11. Wang, Z. et al. Targeting notch to eradicate pancreatic cancer stem cells for cancer therapy. Anticancer Res. 31, 1105–1113 (2011).
12. Sarkar, S. et al. Oxidative inhibition of Hsp90 disrupts the super-chaperone complex and attenuates pancreatic adenocarcinoma in vitro and in vivo. Int. J. Cancer 132, 695–706 (2013).
13. Sarkar, S., Mandal, C., Sangwan, R. & Mandal, C. Coupling G2/M arrest to the Wnt/β-catenin pathway restrains pancreatic adenocarcinoma. Endocr. Relat. Cancer 21, 113–125 (2014).
14. Gialoganglioside GD3-synthase over expression inhibits survival and angiogenesis of pancreatic cancer cells through cell cycle arrest at S-phase and disruption of integrin-β1-mediated anchorage. Int. J. Biochem. Cell Biol. 53, 162–173 (2014).
15. McGuigan Andrew, Kelly Paul , Turkington Richard C, Jones Claire, Coleman Helen G,   McCain R Stephen. Pancreatic cancer: A review of clinical diagnosis, epidemiology, treatment and outcomes. World J Gastroenterol. 2018 Nov 21; 24(43): 4846–4861.
16. Ottenhof NA, de Wilde RF, Maitra A, Hruban RH, Offerhaus GJ. Molecular characteristics of pancreatic ductal adenocarcinoma. Patholog Res Int. 2011 Mar 27;2011:620601.
17. Ryan David P, Hong Theodore S., Bardeesy   Nabeel. Pancreatic Adenocarcinoma. N Engl J Med 2014;371:1039-49.
18. Bardeesy Nabeel, DePinho Ronald A. Pancreatic cancer biology and genetics. Nature Reviews Cancer volume 2, pages897–909(2002)
19. Orth M, Metzger P, Gerum S, Mayerle J, Schneider G, Belka C, Schnurr M, Lauber K. Pancreatic ductal adenocarcinoma: biological hallmarks, current status, and future perspectives of combined modality treatment approaches. Radiat Oncol. 2019 Aug 8;14(1):141.
20. Raimondi S, Lowenfels AB, Morselli-Labate AM, Maisonneuve P, Pezzilli R. Pancreatic cancer in chronic pancreatitis; aetiology, incidence, and early detection. Best Pract Res Clin Gastroenterol. 2010 Jun;24(3):349-58.
21. Carlo Claudia Di, Brandi Jessica, Cecconi Daniela. Pancreatic cancer stem cells: Perspectives on potential therapeutic approaches of pancreatic ductal adenocarcinoma. World J Stem Cells 2018 November 26; 10(11): 172-182.
22. Kamisawa Terumi ,Wood Laura D, Itoi Takao,Takaori Kyoichi. Pancreatic cancer. Lancet 2016; 388: 73–85.
23. Rao Chinthalapally V,   Mohammed Altaf.New insights into pancreatic cancer stem cells. World J Stem Cells. 2015 Apr 26; 7(3): 547–555.
24. Lee Cheong J. , Dosch Joseph , Simeone Diane M.Pancreatic Cancer Stem Cells. Clinical Oncology 26, no. 17 (2008) 2806-2812.
25. Ercan G, Karlitepe A, Ozpolat B.Pancreatic Cancer Stem Cells and Therapeutic Approaches. Anticancer Res. 2017 Jun;37(6):2761-2775.
26. Huang HC, Mallidi S, Liu J, Chiang CT, Mai Z, Goldschmidt R, Ebrahim-Zadeh N, Rizvi I, Hasan T. Photodynamic Therapy Synergizes with Irinotecan to Overcome Compensatory Mechanisms and Improve Treatment Outcomes in Pancreatic Cancer. Cancer Res. 2016 Mar 1;76(5):1066-77.
27. Freelove R, Walling AD. Pancreatic cancer: diagnosis and management. Am Fam Physician. 2006 Feb 1;73(3):485-92.
28. Oberstein Paul E., Kenneth P. Olive. Pancreatic cancer: why is it so hard to treat? Therap Adv Gastroenterol. 2013 Jul; 6(4): 321–337.
29. Gillen Sonja, Schuster Tibor , Büschenfelde Christian Meyer zum, Friess Helmut, Kleeff Jörg. Preoperative/Neoadjuvant Therapy in Pancreatic Cancer: A Systematic Review and Meta-analysis of Response and Resection Percentages. PLoS Med. 2010 Apr; 7(4): e1000267.
30. Krzyzanowska MK, Weeks JC, Earle CC. Treatment of locally advanced pancreatic cancer in the real world: population-based practices and effectiveness. J Clin Oncol. 2003 Sep 15;21(18):3409-14.
31. Lim JE, Chien MW, Earle CC. Prognostic factors following curative resection for pancreatic adenocarcinoma: a population-based, linked database analysis of 396 patients. Ann Surg. 2003 Jan;237(1):74-85.
32. Sultana A, Smith CT, Cunningham D, Starling N, Neoptolemos JP, Ghaneh P. Meta-analyses of chemotherapy for locally advanced and metastatic pancreatic cancer. J Clin Oncol. 2007 Jun 20;25(18):2607-15.

33. Schauer Roland. Sialic ACIDS: Metabolism of O-acetyl groups. Methods in Enzymology 1987 (138); 611-626.
34. Muchmore EA, Milewski M, Varki A, Diaz S. Biosynthesis of N-glycolyneuraminic acid. The primary site of hydroxylation of N-acetylneuraminic acid is the cytosolic sugar nucleotide pool. J Biol Chem. 1989 Dec 5;264(34):20216-23.
35. Myers RW, Lee RT, Lee YC, Thomas GH, Reynolds LW, Uchida Y. The synthesis of 4-methylumbelliferyl alpha-ketoside of N-acetylneuraminic acid and its use in a fluorometric assay for neuraminidase. Anal Biochem. 1980 Jan 1;101(1):166-74.
36. Higa HH, Paulson JC. Sialylation of glycoprotein oligosaccharides with N-acetyl-, N-glycolyl-, and N-O-diacetylneuraminic acids. J Biol Chem. 1985 Jul 25;260(15):8838-49.
37. Ulloa, F. & Real, F. X. Differential distribution of sialic acid in α2, 3 and α2, 6 linkages in the apical membrane of cultured epithelial cells and tissues. J.Histochem. Cytochem. 49, 501–509 (2001).
38. Bassagañas, S., Pérez-Garay, M. & Peracaula, R. Cell surface sialic acid modulates extracellular matrix adhesion and migration in pancreatic adenocarcinoma cells. Pancreas 43, 109–117 (2014).
39. Monti, E. et al. Sialidases in vertebrates. A family of enzymes tailored for several cell functions. Adv. Carbohydr. Chem. Biochem. 64, 403–479 (2010).
40. Mandal, C. Regulation of O-acetylation of sialic acids by sialate-Oacetyltransferase and sialate-O-acetylesterase activities in childhood acute lymphoblastic leukemia. Glycobiology 22, 70–83 (2012).
41. Mondal, S., Chandra, S. & Mandal, C. Elevated mRNA level of hST6Gal I and hST3Gal V positively correlates with the high risk of pediatric acute leukemia. Leuk. Res. 34, 463–470 (2010).
42. Varki A, Cummings RD, Esko JD. Essentials of Glycobiology. 2nd edition Cold Spring Harbor (NY): Cold Spring Harbor Laboratory Press; 2009.
43. Zhou X, Yang G, Guan F. Biological Functions and Analytical Strategies of Sialic Acids in Tumor. Cells. 2020 Jan 22;9(2).
44.Pang Q, Han H, Liu X, Wang Z, Liang Q, Hou J, Qi Q, Wang Q. In vivo evolutionary engineering of riboswitch with high-threshold for N-acetylneuraminic acid production. Metab Eng. 2020 Jan 16;59:36-43.
45. Kelm S1, Schauer R. Sialic acids in molecular and cellular interactions. Int Rev Cytol. 1997;175:137-240.
46. Varki NM1, Varki A. Diversity in cell surface sialic acid presentations: implications for biology and disease. Lab Invest. 2007 Sep;87(9):851-7. Epub 2007 Jul 16.
47. Liu YC, Yen HY, Chen CY, Chen CH, Cheng PF, et al. Sialylation and fucosylation of epidermal growth factor receptor suppress its dimerization and activation in lung cancer cells. Proc Natl Acad Sci U S A. 2011 Jul 12;108(28):11332-7. doi: 10.1073/pnas.1107385108. Epub 2011 Jun 27.
48. Baskakov IV, Katorcha E. Multifaceted Role of Sialylation in Prion Diseases. Front Neurosci. 2016 Aug 8;10:358. doi: 10.3389/fnins.2016.00358. eCollection 2016.
49. Varki A. Sialic acids in human health and disease. Trends Mol Med. 2008 Aug;14(8):351-60. doi: 10.1016/j.molmed.2008.06.002. Epub 2008 Jul 6.
50. Schultz MJ, Swindall AF, Bellis SL. Regulation of the metastatic cell phenotype by sialylated glycans. Cancer Metastasis Rev. 2012 Dec;31(3-4):501-18. doi: 10.1007/s10555-012-9359-7.
51. Schauer R. Sialic acids as regulators of molecular and cellular interactions. Curr Opin Struct Biol. 2009 Oct;19(5):507-14. doi: 10.1016/j.sbi.2009.06.003. Epub 2009 Aug 19.
52. Schwab I, Nimmerjahn F. Role of sialylation in the anti-inflammatory activity of intravenous immunoglobulin - F(ab')₂ versus Fc sialylation. Clin Exp Immunol. 2014 Dec;178 Suppl 1:97-9. doi: 10.1111/cei.12527.
53. Kelm S, Schauer R, Manuguerra JC, Gross HJ, Crocker PR Modifications of cell surface sialic acids modulate cell adhesion mediated by sialoadhesin and CD22. Glycoconj J. 1994 Dec;11(6):576-85.
54. Mandal, C. et al. High level of sialate-O-acetyltransferase activity in lymphoblasts of childhood acute lymphoblastic leukaemia (ALL): enzyme characterization and correlation with disease status. Glycoconj. J. 26, 57–73 (2009).
55. Glavey, S. V. et al. The sialyltransferase ST3GAL6 inflfluences homing and survival in multiple myeloma. Blood 124, 1765–1776 (2014).
56. Harvey, B. E. et al. Sialyltransferase activity and hepatic tumor growth in a nude mouse model of colorectal cancer metastases. Cancer Res. 52, 1775–1779 (1992).
57. Zhao, Y. et al. α2,6-Sialylation mediates hepatocellular carcinoma growth in vitro and in vivo by targeting the Wnt/β-catenin pathway. Oncogenesis 6, e343 (2017).
58. Cao, Y., Merling, A., Crocker, P. R., Keller, R. & Schwartz-Albiez, R. Differential expression of beta-galactosidealpha2,6 sialyltransferase and sialoglycans in normal and cirrhotic liver and hepatocellular carcinoma. Lab. Invest. 82, 1515–1524 (2002).
59.Bassagañas, S. et al. Pancreatic cancer cell glycosylation regulates cell adhesion and invasion through the modulation of α2β1 integrin and E-cadherin function. PLoS ONE 9, e98595 (2014).
60 Hsieh, C.-C. et al. Elevation of β-galactoside α2, 6-sialyltransferase 1 in a fructose- responsive manner promotes pancreatic cancer metastasis. Oncotarget 8, 7691–7709 (2016).
61. Pérez-Garay, M. et al. α2,3-Sialyltransferase ST3Gal IV promotes migration and metastasis in pancreatic adenocarcinoma cells and tends to be highly expressed in pancreatic adenocarcinoma tissues. Int. J. Biochem. Cell Biol. 45, 1748–1757 (2013).
62. Miyagi T, Yamaguchi K. Mammalian sialidases: physiological and pathological roles in cellular functions. Glycobiology. 2012 Jul;22(7):880-96.
63. Monti E, Preti A, Venerando B, Borsani G. Recent development in mammalian sialidase molecular biology. Neurochem Res. 2002 Aug;27(7-8):649-63.
64. Monti E, Bonten E, D'Azzo A, Bresciani R, Venerando B, Borsani G, Schauer R, Tettamanti G. Sialidases in vertebrates: a family of enzymes tailored for several cell functions. Adv Carbohydr Chem Biochem. 2010;64:403-79.
65. Monti E, Miyagi T. Structure and Function of Mammalian Sialidases. Top Curr Chem. 2015;366:183-208.
66. Miyagi T. Aberrant expression of sialidase and cancer progression. Proc Jpn Acad Ser B Phys Biol Sci. 2008;84(10):407-18.
67. Videira PA, Correia M, Malagolini N, Crespo HJ, Ligeiro D, Calais FM, Trindade H, Dall'Olio F. ST3Gal.I sialyltransferase relevance in bladder cancer tissues and cell lines. BMC Cancer. 2009 Oct 7;9:357. doi: 10.1186/1471-2407-9-357.

68. Harduin-Lepers A, Krzewinski-Recchi MA, Colomb F, Foulquier F, Groux-Degroote S, Delannoy P. Sialyltransferases functions in cancers. Front Biosci (Elite Ed). 2012 Jan 1;4:499-515.
69. Chen JY, Tang YA, Huang SM, Juan HF, Wu LW, Sun YC et. al. A novel sialyltransferase inhibitor suppresses FAK/paxillin signaling and cancer angiogenesis and metastasis pathways. Cancer Res. 2011 Jan 15;71(2):473-83.
70. Murugaesu N, Iravani M, van Weverwijk A, Ivetic A, Johnson DA, Antonopoulos A. et. al. An in vivo functional screen identifies ST6GalNAc2 sialyltransferase as a breast cancer metastasis suppressor. Cancer Discov. 2014 Mar;4(3):304-17.
71. Pérez-Garay M, Arteta B, Pagès L, de Llorens R, de Bolòs C, Vidal-Vanaclocha F, Peracaula R. alpha2,3-sialyltransferase ST3Gal III modulates pancreatic cancer cell motility and adhesion in vitro and enhances its metastatic potential in vivo. PLoS One. 2010 Sep 1;5(9).
72. Lee M, Lee HJ, Bae S, Lee YS. Protein sialylation by sialyltransferase involves radiation resistance. Mol Cancer Res. 2008 Aug;6(8):1316-25.
73. Glavey SV, Manier S, Natoni A, Sacco A, Moschetta M, Reagan MR et. al. The sialyltransferase ST3GAL6 influences homing and survival in multiple myeloma. Blood. 2014 Sep 11;124(11):1765-76.
74. Jun L, Yuanshu W, Yanying X, Zhongfa X, Jian Y, Fengling W. et. al. Altered mRNA expressions of sialyltransferases in human gastric cancer tissues. Med Oncol. 2012 Mar;29(1):84-90.
75. Lu J, Gu J. Significance of β-Galactoside α2,6 Sialyltranferase 1 in Cancers. Molecules. 2015 Apr 24;20(5):7509-27.
76. Burchell, J.; Poulsom, R.; Hanby, A.; Whitehouse, C.; Cooper, L.; Clausen, H.; et.al. An alpha2,3 sialyltransferase (ST3Gal I) is elevated in primary breast carcinomas. Glycobiology 1999, 9, 1307–1311.
77. Videira, P.A.; Correia, M.; Malagolini, N.; Crespo, H.J.; Ligeiro, D.; Calais, F.M.; Trindade, H.; Dall'Olio, F. ST3Gal.I sialyltransferase relevance in bladder cancer tissues and cell lines. BMC Cancer 2009, 9, 357.
78. Kudo, T.; Ikehara, Y.; Togayachi, A.; Morozumi, K.; Watanabe, M.; Nakamura, M.; Nishihara, S.; Narimatsu, H. Up-regulation of a set of glycosyltransferase genes in human colorectal cancer. Lab. Investig. 1998, 78, 797–811.
79. Hatano, K.; Miyamoto, Y.; Mori, M.; Nimura, K.; Nakai, Y.; Nonomura, N.; Kaneda, Y. Androgen-regulated transcriptional control of sialyltransferases in prostate cancer cells. PLoS ONE 2012, 7, e31234
80. Perez-Garay, M.; Arteta, B.; Pages, L.; de Llorens, R.; de Bolos, C.; Vidal-Vanaclocha, F.; Peracaula, R. alpha2,3-sialyltransferase ST3Gal III modulates pancreatic cancer cell motility and adhesion in vitro and enhances its metastatic potential in vivo. PLoS ONE 2010, 5, e12524.
81. Gretschel, S.; Haensch, W.; Schlag, P.M.; Kemmner, W. Clinical relevance of sialyltransferasesST6GAL-I and ST3GAL-III in gastric cancer. Oncology 2003, 65, 139–145.
Molecules 2015, 20 7520.
82. Jin, X.L.; Zheng, S.S.; Wang, B.S.; Chen, H.L. Correlation of glycosyltransferases mRNA expression in extrahepatic bile duct carcinoma with clinical pathological characteristics. Hepatobiliary Pancreat. Dis. Int. 2004, 3, 292–295.
83. Wang, P.H.; Li, Y.F.; Juang, C.M.; Lee, Y.R.; Chao, H.T.; Ng, H.T.; Tsai, Y.C.; Yuan, C.C. Expression of sialyltransferase family members in cervix squamous cell carcinoma correlates with lymph node metastasis. Gynecol. Oncol. 2002, 86, 45–52.
84. Gomes, C.; Osorio, H.; Pinto, M.T.; Campos, D.; Oliveira, M.J.; Reis, C.A. Expression of ST3GAL4 leads to SLe(x) expression and induces c-Met activation and an invasive phenotype in gastric carcinoma cells. PLoS ONE 2013, 8, e66737.
85. Saito, S.; Yamashita, S.; Endoh, M.; Yamato, T.; Hoshi, S.; Ohyama, C.; Watanabe, R.; Ito, A.; Satoh, M.; Wada, T.; et al. Clinical significance of ST3Gal IV expression in human renal cell carcinoma. Oncol. Rep. 2002, 9, 1251–1255.
86. Mondal, S.; Chandra, S.; Mandal, C. Elevated mRNA level of hST6Gal I and hST3Gal V positively correlates with the high risk of pediatric acute leukemia. Leuk. Res. 2010, 34, 463–470.
87. Recchi, M.A.; Hebbar, M.; Hornez, L.; Harduin-Lepers, A.; Peyrat, J.P.; Delannoy, P. Multiplex reverse transcription polymerase chain reaction assessment of sialyltransferase expression in human breast cancer. Cancer Res. 1998, 58, 4066–4070.
88. Dall'Olio, F.; Malagolini, N.; di Stefano, G.; Minni, F.; Marrano, D.; Serafini-Cessi, F. Increased CMP-NeuAc:Gal beta 1,4GlcNAc-R alpha 2,6 sialyltransferase activity in human colorectal cancer. Int. J. Cancer 1989, 44, 434–439.
89. Skacel, P.O.; Edwards, A.J.; Harrison, C.T.; Watkins, W.M. Enzymic control of the expression of the X determinant (CD15) in human myeloid cells during maturation: The regulatory role of 6-sialyltransferase. Blood 1991, 78, 1452–1460.
90. Fukushima, K.; Hara-Kuge, S.; Seko, A.; Ikehara, Y.; Yamashita, K. Elevation of alpha2-->6 sialyltransferase and alpha1-->2 fucosyltransferase activities in human choriocarcinoma. Cancer Res. 1998, 58, 4301–4306.
91. Wang, P.H.; Li, Y.F.; Juang, C.M.; Lee, Y.R.; Chao, H.T.; Tsai, Y.C.; Yuan, C.C. Altered mRNA expression of sialyltransferase in squamous cell carcinomas of the cervix. Gynecol. Oncol. 2001, 83, 121–127.
92. Kaneko, Y.; Yamamoto, H.; Kersey, D.S.; Colley, K.J.; Leestma, J.E.; Moskal, J.R. The expression of Gal beta 1,4GlcNAc alpha 2,6 sialyltransferase and alpha 2,6-linked sialoglycoconjugates in human brain tumors. Acta Neuropathol. 1996, 91, 284–292.
93. Zhao, Y.; Li, Y.; Ma, H.; Dong, W.; Zhou, H.; Song, X.; Zhang, J.; Jia, L. Modification of sialylation mediates the invasive properties and chemosensitivity of human hepatocellular carcinoma. Mol. Cell. Proteomics 2014, 13, 520–536.
94. Dall'Olio, F.; Trere, D. Expression of alpha 2,6-sialylated sugar chains in normal and neoplastic colon tissues. Detection by digoxigenin-conjugated Sambucus nigra agglutinin. Eur. J. Histochem. 1993, 37, 257–265.
95. Sata, T.; Roth, J.; Zuber, C.; Stamm, B.; Heitz, P.U. Expression of alpha 2,6-linked sialic acid residues in neoplastic but not in normal human colonic mucosa. A lectin-gold cytochemical study with Sambucus nigra and Maackia amurensis lectins. Am. J. Pathol. 1991, 139, 1435–1448.
96. Dall'Olio, F.; Chiricolo, M.; D'Errico, A.; Gruppioni, E.; Altimari, A.; Fiorentino, M.; Grigioni, W.F. Expression of beta-galactoside alpha2,6 sialyltransferase and of alpha2,6-sialylated glycoconjugates in normal human liver, hepatocarcinoma, and cirrhosis. Glycobiology 2004, 14, 39–49.
97. Julien, S.; Adriaenssens, E.; Ottenberg, K.; Furlan, A.; Courtand, G.; Vercoutter-Edouart, A.S.; Hanisch, F.G.; Delannoy, P.; Le Bourhis, X. ST6GalNAc I expression in MDA-MB-231 breast cancer cells greatly modifies their O-glycosylation pattern and enhances their tumourigenicity.Glycobiology 2006, 16, 54–64.

98. Marcos, N.T.; Pinho, S.; Grandela, C.; Cruz, A.; Samyn-Petit, B.; Harduin-Lepers, A.; Almeida, R.; Silva, F.; Morais, V.; Costa, J.; et al. Role of the human ST6GalNAc-I and ST6GalNAc-II in the synthesis of the cancer-associated sialyl-Tn antigen. Cancer Res. 2004, 64, 7050–7057.
99. Vázquez-Martín, C.; Cuevas, E.; Gil-Martín, E.; Fernández-Briera, A. Correlation Analysis between Tumorous Associated Antigen Sialyl-Tn Expression and ST6GalNAc I Activity in Human Colon Adenocarcinoma. Oncology 2004, 67, 159–165.
100. Pinho, S.; Marcos, N.T.; Ferreira, B.; Carvalho, A.S.; Oliveira, M.J.; Santos-Silva, F.; Harduin-Lepers, A.; Reis, C.A. Biological significance of cancer-associated sialyl-Tn antigen: Modulation of malignant phenotype in gastric carcinoma cells. Cancer Lett. 2007, 249, 157–170.
101. Schneider, F.; Kemmner, W.; Haensch, W.; Franke, G.; Gretschel, S.; Karsten, U.; Schlag, P.M. Overexpression of sialyltransferase CMP-sialic acid: Galbeta1,3GalNAc-R alpha6-Sialyltransferase is related to poor patient survival in human colorectal carcinomas. Cancer Res. 2001, 61, 4605–4611.
102. Bos, P.D.; Zhang, X.H.F.; Nadal, C.; Shu, W.P.; Gomis, R.R.; Nguyen, D.X.; Minn, A.J.; van de Vijver, M.J.; Gerald, W.L.; Foekens, J.A.; et al. Genes that mediate breast cancer metastasis to the brain. Nature 2009, 459, 1005–1009.
103. Tsuchida, A.; Okajima, T.; Furukawa, K.; Ando, T.; Ishida, H.; Yoshida, A.; Nakamura, Y.; Kannagi, R.; Kiso, M.; Furukawa, K. Synthesis of disialyl Lewis a (Le(a)) structure in colon cancer cell lines by a sialyltransferase, ST6GalNAc VI, responsible for the synthesis of alpha-series gangliosides. J. Biol. Chem. 2003, 278, 22787–22794.
104. Miyazaki, K.; Ohmori, K.; Izawa, M.; Koike, T.; Kumamoto, K.; Furukawa, K.; Ando, T.; Kiso, M.;Yamaji, T.; Hashimoto, Y.; et al. Loss of disialyl Lewis(a), the ligand for lymphocyte inhibitory receptor sialic acid-binding immunoglobulin-like lectin-7 (Siglec-7) associated with increased sialyl Lewis(a) expression on human colon cancers. Cancer Res. 2004, 64, 4498–4505.
105. Steenackers, A.; Vanbeselaere, J.; Cazet, A.; Bobowski, M.; Rombouts, Y.; Colomb, F.; Le Bourhis, X.; Guerardel, Y.; Delannoy, P. Accumulation of unusual gangliosides G(Q3) and G(P3) in breast cancer cells expressing the G(D3) synthase. Molecules 2012, 17, 9559–9572.
106. Kim, S.J.; Chung, T.W.; Jin, U.H.; Suh, S.J.; Lee, Y.C.; Kim, C.H. Molecular mechanisms involved in transcriptional activation of the human Sia-alpha2,3-Gal-beta1,4-GlcNAc-R: Alpha2,8-sialyltransferase (hST8Sia III) gene induced by KCl in human glioblastoma cells.Biochem. Biophys. Res. Commun. 2006, 344, 1057–1064.
107. Miyagi T, Takahashi K, Hata K, Shiozaki K, Yamaguchi Y. Sialidase significance for cancer progression. Glycoconj J. 2012 Dec;29(8-9):567-77.
108. Glanz VY, Myasoedova VA, Grechko AV, Orekhov AN. Sialidase activity in human pathologies.Eur J Pharmacol. 2019 Jan 5;842:345-350.
109. Schwerdtfeger SM, Melzig MF. Sialidases in biological systems. Pharmazie. 2010 Aug;65(8):551-61.
110. Miyagi T, Wada T, Yamaguchi K, Shiozaki K, Sato I, Kakugawa Y, Yamanami H, Fujiya T.Human sialidase as a cancer marker. Proteomics. 2008 Aug;8(16):3303-11.
111. D'Azzo A, Hoogeveen A, Reuser AJ, Robinson D, Galjaard H. 1982.Molecular defect in combined beta-galactosidase and neuraminidase defi-ciency in man. Proc Natl Acad Sci USA. 79:4535–4539.
112. Bonten E, van der Spoel A, Fornerod M, Grosveld G, d'Azzo A. 1996.Characterization of human lysosomal neuraminidase defines the molecular basis of the metabolic storage disorder sialidosis. Genes Dev.10:3156–3169.
113. Hinek A, Pshezhetsky AV, von Itzstein M, Starcher B. 2006. Lysosomal sialidase (neuraminidase-1) is targeted to the cell surface in a multiproteinc omplex that facilitates elastic fiber assembly. J Biol Chem.281:3698–3710.
114. Jayanth P, Amith SR, Gee K, Szewczuk MR. 2010. Neu1 sialidase and matrixmetalloproteinase-9 cross-talk is essential for neurotrophin activation of Trk receptors and cellular signaling. Cell Signal. 22:1193–1205.
115. Katoh S, Maeda S, Fukuoka H, Wada T, Moriya S, Mori A, Yamaguchi K,Senda S, Miyagi T. 2010. A crucial role of sialidase Neu1 in hyaluronan receptor function of CD44 in T helper type 2-mediated airway inflammation of murine acute asthmatic model. Clin Exp Immunol. 161:233–241.
116. Katoh S, Miyagi T, Taniguchi H, Matsubara Y, Kadota J, Tominaga A,Kincade PW, Matsukura S, Kohno S. 1999. Cutting edge: An inducible sialidase regulates the hyaluronic acid binding ability of CD44-bearing human monocytes. J Immunol. 162:5058–5061.
117. Hou G, Liu G, Yang Y, Li Y, Yuan S, Zhao L et.al. Neuraminidase 1 (NEU1) promotes proliferation and migration as a diagnostic and prognostic biomarker of hepatocellular carcinoma. Oncotarget. 2016 Oct 4;7(40):64957-64966.
118. Gilmour AM, Abdulkhalek S, Cheng TS, Alghamdi F, Jayanth P, O'Shea LK, et.al. A novel epidermal growth factor receptor-signaling platform and its targeted translation in pancreatic cancer. Cell Signal. 2013 Dec;25(12):2587-603.
119. Chavas LM, Tringali C, Fusi P, Venerando B, Tettamanti G, Kato R, et. al. Crystal structure of the human cytosolic sialidase Neu2. Evidence for the dynamic nature of substrate recognition. J Biol Chem. 2005 Jan 7;280(1):469-75.
120. Fanzani, A., Colombo, F., Giuliani, R., Preti, A. & Marchesini, S. Cytosolic sialidase Neu2 upregulation during PC12 cells differentiation. FEBS Lett. (2004) 566, 178–182.
121. Fanzani, A. et al. Overexpression of cytosolic sialidase Neu2 induces myoblast differentiation in C2C12 cells. FEBS Lett. (2003) 547, 183–188.
122. Stoppani E, Rossi S, Marchesini S, Preti A, Fanzani A. 2009. Defective myogenic differentiation of human rhabdomyosarcoma cells is characterized by sialidase Neu2 loss of expression. Cell Biol Int. 33:1020–1025.
123. Tringali, C. et al. Expression of sialidase Neu2 in leukemic K562 cells induces apoptosis by impairing Bcr-Abl/Src kinases signaling. J. Biol. Chem. 282,14364–14372 (2007).
124. Tokuyama, S. et al. Suppression of pulmonary metastasis in murine B16 melanoma cells by transfection of a sialidase cDNA. Int. J. Cancer (1997) 73, 410–415.
125. Sawada, M. et al. Reduced sialidase expression in highly metastatic variants of mouse colon adenocarcinoma 26 and retardation of their metastatic ability by sialidase overexpression. Int. J. Cancer (2002) 97, 180–185.
126. Tokuyama S, Moriya S, Taniguchi S, Yasui A, Miyazaki J, Orikasa S, Miyagi T. Suppression of pulmonary metastasis in murine B16 melanoma cells by transfection of a sialidase cDNA. Int J Cancer. 1997 Nov 4;73(3):410-5.

127. Meuillet EJ, Kroes R, Yamamoto H, Warner TG, Ferrari J, Mania-Farnell B. et.al. Sialidase gene transfection enhances epidermal growth factor receptor activity in an epidermoid carcinoma cell line, A431. Cancer Res. 1999 59:234–240.
128. Yamaguchi K, Koseki K, Shiozaki M, Shimada Y, Wada T, Miyagi T. 2010. Regulation of plasma-membrane-associated sialidase NEU3 gene by Sp1/Sp3 transcription factors. Biochem J. 430:107–117.
129. Zanchetti G, Colombi P, Manzoni M, Anastasia L, Caimi L, Borsani G et al. . Sialidase NEU3 is a peripheral membrane protein localized on the cell surface and in endosomal structures. Biochem J. 2007 408:211–219.
130. Forcella M, Oldani M, Epistolio S, Freguia S, Monti E, Fusi P, Frattini M. Non-small cell lung cancer (NSCLC), EGFR downstream pathway activation and TKI targeted therapies sensitivity: Effect of the plasma membrane-associated NEU3. PLoS One. 2017 Oct 31;12(10):e0187289.
131. Shiga K, Takahashi K, Sato I, Kato K, Saijo S, Moriya S et. al. Upregulation of sialidase NEU3 in head and neck squamous cell carcinoma associated with lymph node metastasis. Cancer Sci. 2015 Nov;106(11):1544-53.
132. Valaperta R, Chigorno V, Basso L, Prinetti A, Bresciani R, Preti A, Miyagi T, Sonnino S. Plasma membrane production of ceramide from ganglioside GM3 in human fibroblasts. FASEB J. 2006 Jun;20(8):1227-9.
133. Kawamura S, Sato I, Wada T, Yamaguchi K, Li Y, Li D, Zhao X, Ueno S,Aoki H, Tochigi T, et al. . Plasma membrane-associated sialidase (NEU3) regulates progression of prostate cancer to androgen-independent growth through modulation of androgen receptor signaling. Cell Death Differ. 2012 19:170–179.
134. Li X, Zhang L, Shao Y, Liang Z, Shao C, Wang B, Guo B, Li N, Zhao X, Li Y, et al. Effects of a human plasma membrane-associated sialidase siRNA on prostate cancer invasion. Biochem Biophys Res Commun.2011 416:270–276.
135. Mandal C, Tringali C, Mondal S, Anastasia L, Chandra S, Venerando B, Mandal C. Down regulation of membrane-bound Neu3 constitutes a new potential marker for childhood acute lymphoblastic leukemia and induces apoptosis suppression of neoplastic cells. Int J Cancer. 2010 Jan 15;126(2):337-49.
136. Yamanami H, Shiozaki K, Wada T, Yamaguchi K, Uemura T, Kakugawa Y et.al. Down-regulation of sialidase NEU4 may contribute to invasive properties of human colon cancers. Cancer Sci. 2007 Mar;98(3):299-307.
137. Proshin S, Yamaguchi K, Wada T, Miyagi T . Modulation of neuritogenesis by ganglioside-specific sialidase (Neu 3) in human neuroblastoma NB-1 cells. Neurochem Res 2002; 27: 841–846.
138. Tringali C, Cirillo F, Lamorte G, Papini N, Anastasia L, Lupo B et al. NEU4L sialidase overexpression promotes beta-catenin signaling in neuroblastoma cells, enhancing stem-like malignant cell growth. Int J Cancer 2012; 131: 1768–1778.
139. Silvestri I, Testa F, Zappasodi R, Cairo CW, Zhang Y, Lupo B et. al. Sialidase NEU4 is involved in glioblastoma stem cell survival. Cell Death Dis. 2014 Aug 21;5:e1381. doi: 10.1038/cddis.2014.349.

CHAPTER II

Comprehension of the effect of sialidase (Neu2) in modulating Fas activation in pancreatic cancer

2.1 Aim of the study

● Status of mammalian sialidases (lysosomal-Neu1, cytosolic-Neu2, membrane bound Neu3 and luminal Neu4) in in patient samples

● Status of four different mammalian sialidases in pancreatic ductal cancer cell lines (PDAC)

● Modulation of the expression of Neu2 and its role in apoptosis of PDAC cells

● Effect of Neu2 in the regulation of cell cycle

● Deciphering the molecules involved in apoptotic pathways controlled by Neu2

● Detection of cytosolic Neu2 on plasma membrane

● Deciphering linkage-specific sialylation on cell-surface of Neu2-transfected cells

● Association of membrane-bound Neu2 with specific cell surface molecules involved in apoptotic pathway

● Establishment of   Neu2-mediated extrinsic apoptotic pathway

2.2 Summary

Neu2 expression is lowest among other sialidases in different PDAC cells. In also patient tissues lowest expression of Neu2 was found, and a significant strong association with clinicopathological characteristics. Neu2-overexpression caused apoptosis in PDAC cells which was resulted by decreased Bcl2/Bax ratio, activation of several caspases specially caspase 8, a hallmark protein known for extrinsic pathway-mediated apoptosis, with unaffected caspase-9 a main molecule of intrinsic pathway. Several other molecules like Fas/CD95-death receptor, FasL, FADD which are the main drivers of the extrinsic pathway-mediated apoptosis are also up-regulated. Thereby, Neu2 induced extrinsic pathway-mediated apoptosis in PDAC. Interestingly, the enhanced enzyme activity of Neu2-overexpressed cells was found in cytosol as well as on plasma membrane. Membrane bound-Neu2 exhibited enhanced association with Fas causing its desialylation which were confirmed by the decreased association of Fas with SNA (α2,6-sialic acid-binding lectin). Desialylation of α2,6-linked sialic acids (which is a substrate of Neu2) on Fas lead to its activation. Such desialylation possibly responsible for this activation leading to enhanced apoptosis through extrinsic pathway in PDAC cells. Additionally, Neu2-overexpressed PDAC cells demonstrated reduced expression of several cell cycle related molecules like CDK2/CDK4/CDK6, and cyclin-B1/cyclin-E. Taken together, main findings of our study ascertains a novel concept by which the function of Fas/CD95 could be modulated indicating a critical role of upstream Neu2 as a promising target for inducing apoptosis in pancreatic cancer.

2.3 Introduction

More than 90% of pancreatic cancers are pancreatic ductal-adenocarcinoma (PDAC), is fatal due to poor diagnosis and prognosis high metastatic property and drug resistance[1-6.] The multifaceted biological mechanisms remain mostly unknown. Abnormal glycosylation and fucosylation are common features in cancers[7-11]. Hence, these alterations play a significant role in modulating differentiation, signalling, adhesion, invasiveness, metastasis, and apoptosis[12]. Pancreatic cancer cells exhibited higher α2,3- and α2,6-linked sialic acids which mainly affects its higher rate of metastasis[13,14]. Enhanced level of sialic acids depend on the balance of sialic acid modulatory enzymes sialyltransferases and sialidases[15-17]. Elevated levels of the sialyltransferases are common in cancers including PDAC[18-25]. Sialidases behave differently during carcinogenesis[26,27].Mammalian cells have four sialidases namely lysosomal (Neu1), cytosolic (Neu2), membrane bound (Neu3), and luminal (Neu4) differing in their enzymatic property and substrate specificity. The expression of sialidase (Neu2) is either very low or undetectable in most cancers [28-30].

Death receptor Fas (CD95) which stimulates apoptosis is commonly disrupted and implicated in tumour cell survival[31,32]. Both O- and N-linked glycans and α2,6-sialylations of Fas are reported only in colon cancer[33]. The substrate specificity of Neu2 is towards glycoproteins/glycolipids and oligosaccharides.

The relation between sialic acids on Fas and whether Neu2 can play any role in the removal of sialic acids from Fas which leads to its activation in PDAC are not reported. Therefore, we took an attempt to decipher this relation between Neu2 and sialylated Fas in PDAC.

So, here in this study the role of overexpressed-Neu2 on modulation of sialylated-Fas have been investigated in details in pancreatic cancer cells.

2.4 Results

Neu2 is down regulated in human pancreatic cancer tissues

Initially, we compared the status of Neu1/Neu2/Neu3/Neu4 in cancer and adjacent normal tissue specimens by immunohistochemistry (Fig. 2.1A). Optical density score conferred higher Neu1, Neu3 and Neu4 positivity in the tumour tissues (Fig. 2.1B). In contrast, statistically significant low or undetectable expression of Neu2 was observed in all tissues from 20 patients compared to 20 normal adjacent counterparts (Table 2.1A). Interestingly, we observed a strong association of reduced expression of Neu2 with clinicopathological characteristics of these patients. This data suggested that the loss of Neu2 possibly helps higher sialylation status in manifestation of this cancer.

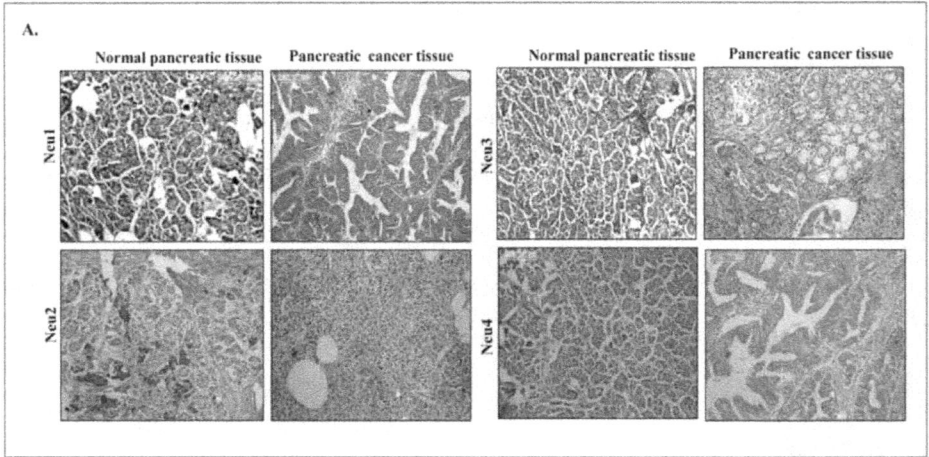

Figure 2.1 (A) The Neu1, Neu2, Neu3, Neu4 protein levels were detected in human pancreatic cancer and normal tissue specimens by immunohistochemistry using respective antibodies. Representative images of pancreatic adenocarcinoma were taken with 20X magnification, showing high positivity for Neu1, Neu3 and Neu4 than normal tissue, poorly differentiated adenocarcinoma showing reduced expression of Neu2 than normal tissue.

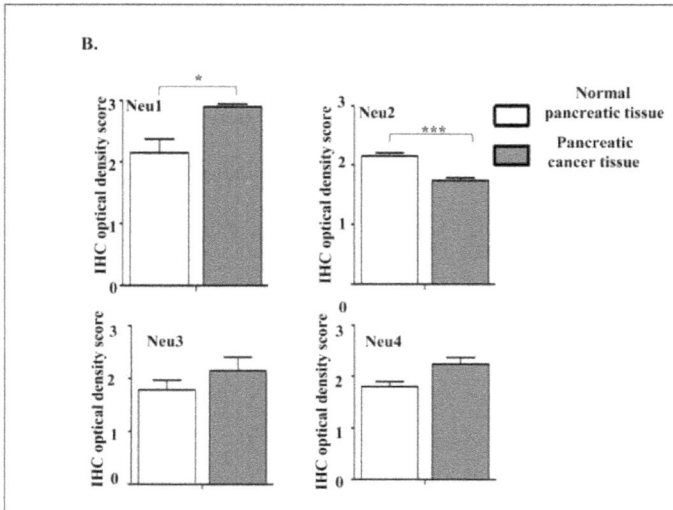

Figure 2.1 (B) Bar graphs represent IHC optical density scores of normal & patient tissue samples for Neu1, Neu2, Neu3 and Neu4 sialidases as measured by ImageJ software.

Table. 2.1A

Association of Neu2 expression with clinicopathological characteristics in patients with pancreatic cancer

Gender		M category	
Male	12	M0	20
Female	8	M1	0
Age	40-85	Surgical Procedure	
Location of tumour		Pancreatoduodenectomy	20
Head, body	20	Histological differentiation	
T category		Well	3
T1	1	Moderately	16
T2	11	Poorly	1
T3	8	Chemotherapy	0
N category		Adjuvant therapy	0
N0	11	Neu2 expression	
N1	9	Neu2 Negative	17
		Neu2 positive	3

Table 2.1B   Mutations in Pancreatic ductal adenocarcinoma (PDAC) cells

Cell Line	K-ras	AKT219q	p16HD	p16Mut	13qLOH	BRCA2 Mut	17pLOH	p53Mut	MKK4HD
MIAPaCa2	12 Cys	-	HD	-	-	-	LOH	248 Trp	-
AsPC1	12 Asp	Ampl.	-	2 bpdel.	LOH	-	LOH	1 bp del.	HD
BxPC3	-	Poss. Ampl.	HD		LOH	-	LOH	220 Cys	-
PANC1	12 Asp	Ampl.	HD		LOH	-	LOH	273 His	-

• MIAPaCa2 is derived from primary tumor, having K-RAS activating mutation, p53 inactivating mutation and   p16 homozygous deletion

- AsPC1 is derived from ascites having K-RAS activating mutation, p53 inactivating mutation, p16 frame shift mutation, Akt amplification and MKK4 homozygous deletion

- BxPC3 is derived from primary tumor, having Akt amplification , p53 inactivating mutation and   p16 homozygous deletion

- PANC1 is derived from primary tumor, having K-RAS activating mutation, p53 inactivating mutation and   p16 homozygous deletion

Real-time PCR analysis of sialidases in these four representatives PDAC cells (Table 2.1B) showed reduced Neu2 expression compared to other three sialidases (Fig. 2.1C). However, MIAPaCa2 and AsPC1 exhibited lowest Neu2 expression among them. Interestingly, they also possess different mutations status. Hence, we have selected these two cells for subsequent study. RT-PCR analysis of all these sialidases also showed similar trend in MIAPaCa2 and AsPC1 (Fig. 2.1D)

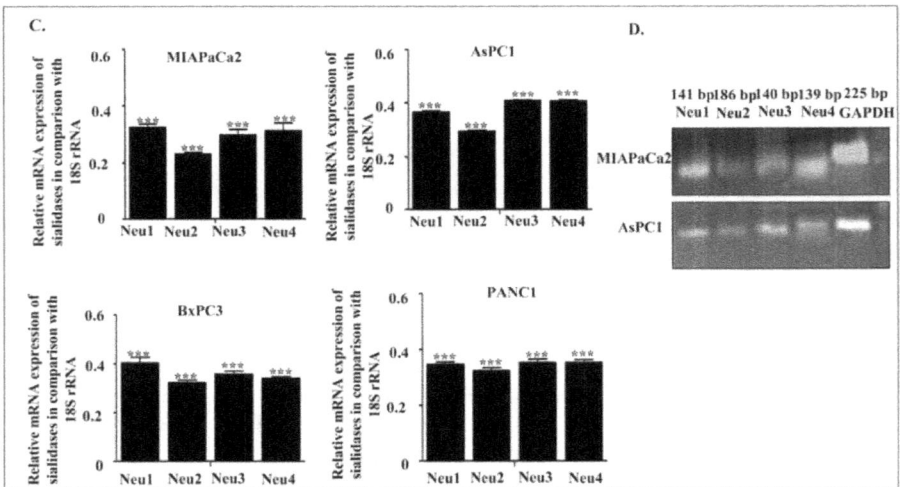

Figure 2.1 (C) Genetic expression of four different sialidases in MIAPaCa2, AsPC1, BxPC3 and PANC1 cells. Relative mRNA expression of Neu1, Neu2, Neu3 and Neu4 was evaluated by real-time PCR analysis. Values are normalized against 18S rRNA expression (n = 3 experiments). (D) Genetic expressions of different sialidases were additionally measured in MIAPaCa2 and AsPC1 cell lines by semi-quantitative RT-PCR. GAPDH was used as loading control.

Accordingly, Neu2 was transfected in MIAPaCa2 and AsPC1. Neu2-transfected cells exhibited higher mRNA expression of Neu2 than mock both by real time PCR (Fig. 2.2A) and RT-PCR (Fig. 2.2B).

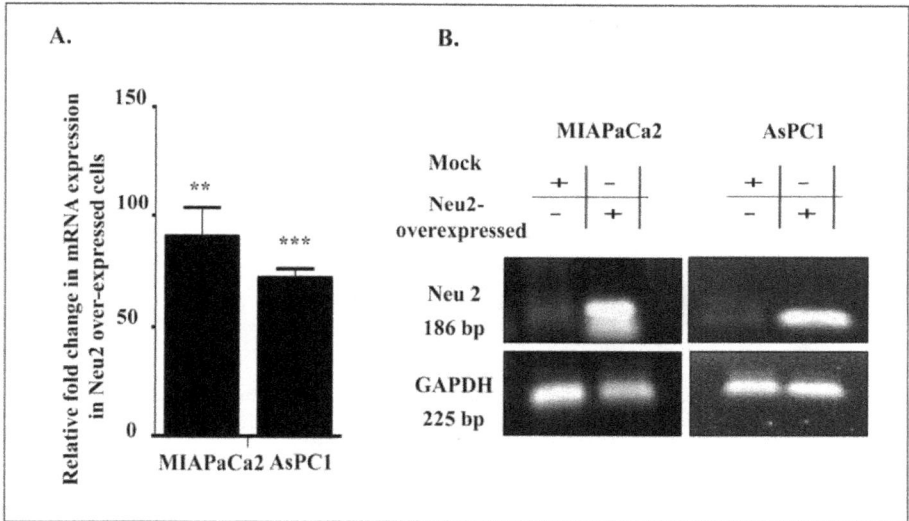

2.2 (A,B) Enhanced Neu2 expression in Neu2-transfected PDAC cells. PDAC cells were transfected with the mock and PcDNA3.1-Neu2 expression vector. Neu2 expression was measured after transfection. Real time and semi-quantitative RT-PCR analysis were done from mock and Neu2-overexpressed cells. Fold change in mRNA expression of Neu2 by real-time PCR analysis in MIAPaCa2, AsPC1 relative to that of mock transfected cells were determined. Values were normalized against 18S rRNA expression (n = 3 experiments). GAPDH was used as loading control for semi-quantitative RT-PCR.

Western blot analysis also revealed enhanced level of Neu2 protein (Fig. 2.2C). However, the expression of Neu1, Neu3 and Neu4 remain unchanged in Neu2-over expressed MIAPaCa2 (Fig. 2.2D) and AsPC1 (Fig. 2.2E).

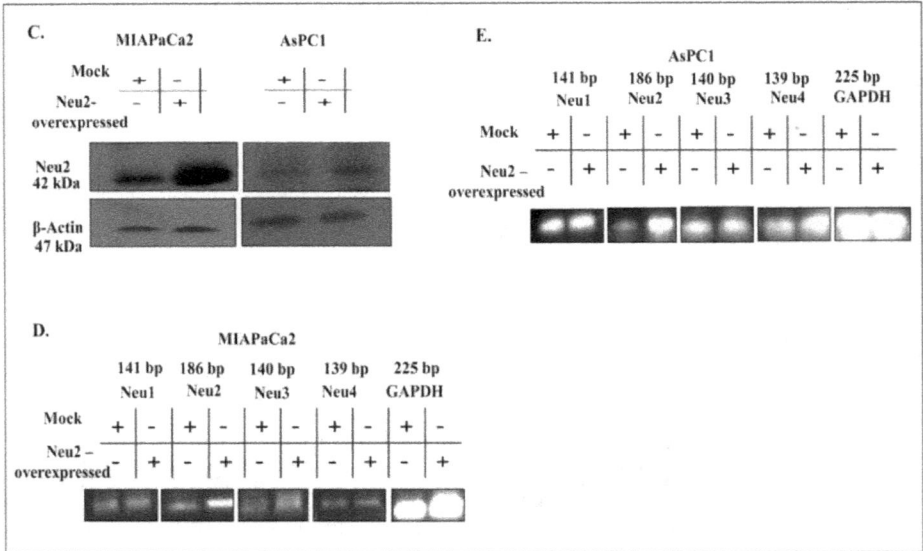

Figure 2.2 (C) Higher level of Neu2 protein in Neu2-transfected MIAPaCa2, AsPC1 cells. Cell lysate from mock and Neu2-overexpressed PDAC cells was used for western blot analysis to determine the status of Neu2 protein. β-actin was used as loading control. (D-E) Genetic expression of different sialidases by RT-PCR in MIAPaCa2 and AsPC1 cells after Neu2-overexpression. GAPDH was used as loading control.

Sialidase activity in Neu2-transfected cells

We measured the sialidase activity both in cytosolic and membrane fractions of Neu2-transfected cells separately at pH 5.5 toward an artificial substrate MU-NeuAc (Fig.2.3 A-D). An increased cytosolic enzyme activity was observed in the Neu2-transfected MIAPaCa2 (0.2414 ± 0.0044 μM/h/mg protein) compared to mock-transfected (0.09842 ± 0.00026 μM/h/mg protein) cells (Fig. 2.3A). Similar trend was found in Neu2-transfected AsPC1 (0.2579 ± 0.019 μM/h/mg protein) compared to mock (0.1048 ± 0.0266 μM/h/mg protein) (Fig.2.3C).

We also found increased level of sialidase activity on membrane in Neu2-over expressed MIAPaCa2 (mock = 0.0340 ± 0.0077 vs. Neu2 = 0.07767 ± 0.0107 μM/h/mg protein) (Fig. 2.3B). Neu2-transfected AsPC1 also exhibited similar pattern; mock = 0.04372 ± 0.0027 vs. Neu2 = 0.09933 ± 0.0108 μM/h/mg protein (Fig. 2.3D). Hence it may be concluded that though Neu2 is a cytosolic enzyme, it also exhibited slightly higher sialidase activity in membrane fraction.

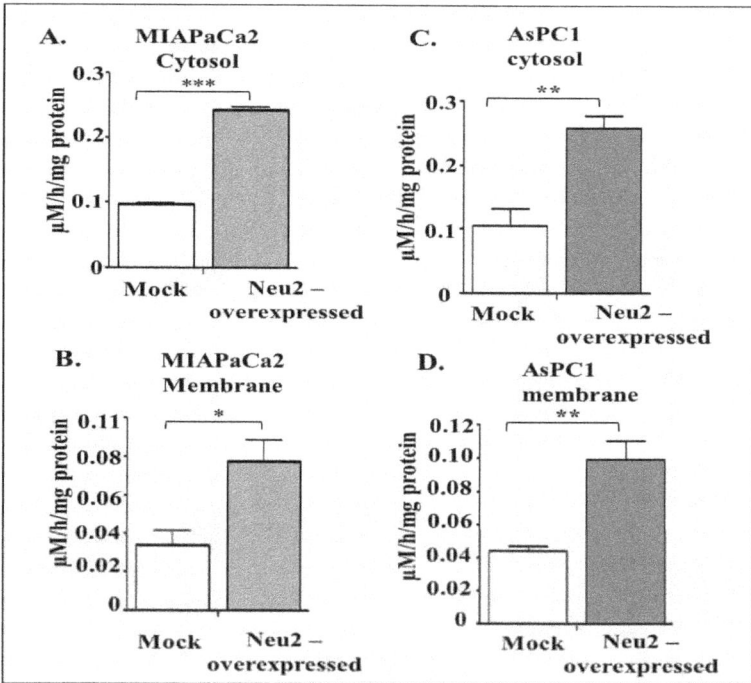

Figure 2.3 (A,C) Enhanced sialidase activity in cytosol of Neu2-overexpressed PDAC cells. The enzyme activity of cytosolic protein (50μg) of Neu2-overexpressed PDAC cells were measured at pH 5.5 using MU-Neu5Ac as substrate by fluorimetric method with excitation at 365 nm and emission at 450 nm. Mock-transfected cells were used for comparison. (B,D) Membrane fractions exhibited higher sialidase activity Neu2-overexpressed PDAC cells. Sialidase activity in 100 μg of protein of the membrane fractions of Neu2-overexpressed MIAPaCa2 cells was determined at pH 5.5 by fluorimetric method

Neu2-over expression inhibits cell proliferation

Next, we checked the growth potential of MIAPaCa2 and AsPC1 due to enhanced-Neu2 activity by MTT assay. The Neu2-transfected cells revealed an impaired proliferation capacity after 3 days of culture in the serum-starved condition which was used as apoptotic stimuli compared to mock. Less number of viable Neu2-over expressed MIAPaCa2 (Fig. 2.4A) and AsPC1 (Fig. 2.4C) cells compared to mock were observed in microscope. The percent of cell viability was significantly reduced by 51.35 ±11.74 and 48.67 ± 0.78 in MIAPaCa2 (Fig. 2.4B) and AsPC1 (Fig. 2.4D) respectively by MTT.

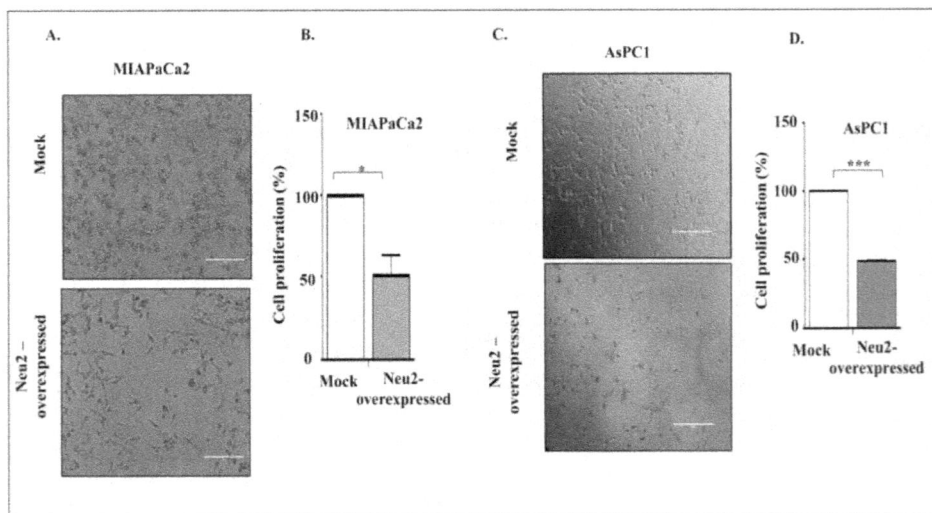

Figure 2.4 (A,C) Neu2-overexpressed MIAPaCa2 and AsPC1 exhibited less cell viability. Mock ad Neu2-overexpressed PDAC cells were visualized by a phase contrast microscope with the magnification of 20X (Evos inverted microscope, Life Technologies). (B,D) Cell viability of mock and Neu2-overexpressed PDAC cells were determined by MTT assay. Cell viability was represented as % proliferation between mock and Neu2-transfected PDAC cells. The data are the means ± S.D. of three different experiments.

Neu2-induced apoptosis is confirmed by annexin V/PI

Since significant cell death was observed in Neu2-transfected cells, we checked the mode of this event after 24h serum starvation. Neu2-overexpression caused surface phosphatidylserine externalization in MIAPaCa2. AnnexinV positivity was 10.90±0.493 compared to 6.47±0.203 in mock-transfected cells illustrating the features of early apoptosis (Fig. 2.5). Neu2-transfected AsPC1 also exhibited higher annexin V positivity.

A substantial number (36.9 ± 1.429) of Neu2-transfected MIAPaCa2 lost membrane integrity and showed late apoptotic bodies as evidenced by both annexin V and PI positivity. AsPC1 also showed a similar trend. Hence it is confirmed that growth-inhibition in Neu2-transfected cells was due to apoptosis.

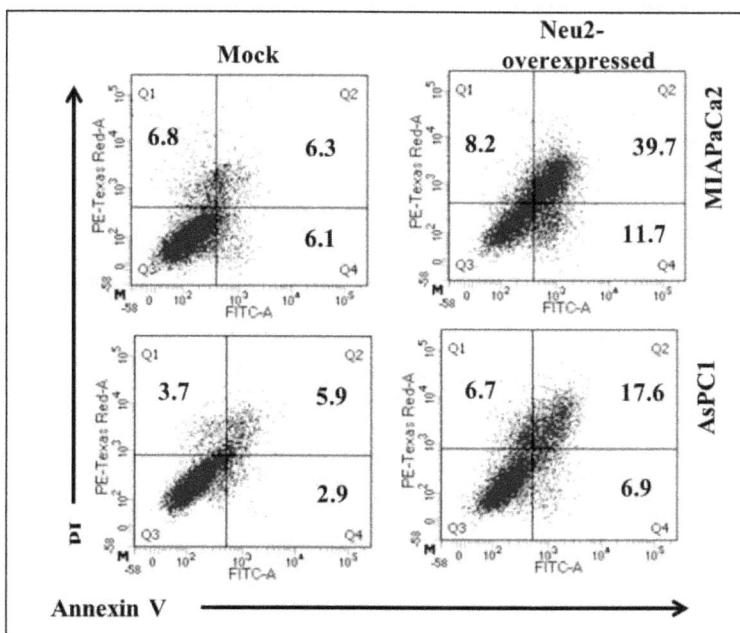

Figure 2.5 Neu2 induces apoptosis in the MIAPaCa2 and AsPC1 cell lines. Effects of Neu2-overexpression on PDAC cells was determined using annexinV–PI staining by flow cytometry. The percentage of apoptosis in Neu2-transfected PDAC cells has been shown in the dot plot. Mock-transfected cells were used as controls.

Neu2-overexpression modulates cell cycle-related proteins

To determine whether growth-inhibition induced by Neu2 was associated with the regulation of cell cycle-related proteins, we checked the status of these molecules both in mock and Neu2-transfected cells by immunoblotting (Fig. 2.6). Neu2-overexpression up-regulated Chk1 and Chk2. Activated Chk1 and Chk2 subsequently led to the reduction of the cyclins and cyclin-dependent kinases. We observed that early G1-cell cycle phase regulatory proteins (CDK4 and CDK6) were down-regulated after Neu2-overexpression. Late G1-phase regulatory proteins (cyclin E and CDK2) were also reduced. Additionally, cyclin B1 involved in the transition of G2 to the M phase was decreased. Modulation of all these proteins suggested that enhanced Neu2 hinders cell growth by impeding different checkpoints, hence it may be stated that as an enzyme it affects the overall cell cycle phases.

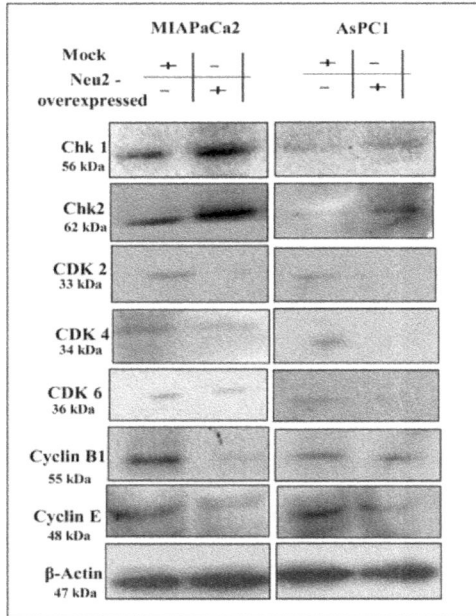

Figure 2.6 Neu2-overexpression modulate cell cycle related proteins in both PDAC cells. Neu2-induced regulation of known molecular mediators of cell cycle in PDAC cells was analyzed by western blot showing upregulation of Chk1, Chk2. Down regulation of CDK2, CDK 4, CDK 6 and cyclin B1 and cyclin E was observed as determined by immunoblot analysis. β-actin was used as loading control

Neu2 induces modulation of anti-apoptotic and pro-apoptotic molecules

We then investigated the probable cause of the observed susceptibility to apoptotic stimuli. We found enhanced mRNA expression of the pro-apoptotic genes (Bax) and effector caspase (caspase 3), but not caspase 9 in Neu2-overexpressed MIAPaCa2 compared to mock-transfected cells after 24h and 48h (Fig. 2.7A).

We also observed higher mRNA level expression of Bax and Cas3 in both MIAPaCa2 (Fig. 2.7B) and AsPC1 (Fig. 2.7C) by real-time PCR analysis after 48h. However, the lower genetic expressions of caspase 9 were observed in both the cells.

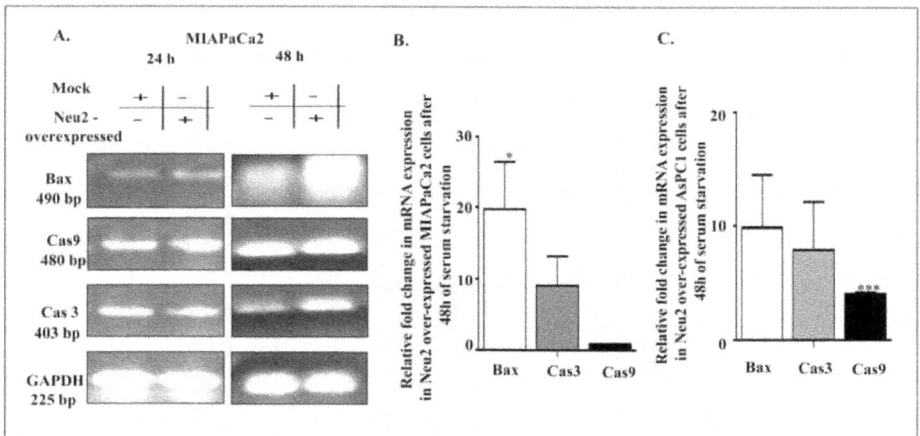

Figure 2.7 (A) MIAPaCa2 cells were transfected and serum starved for 24h and 48h. mRNA expression showed up regulation of pro-apoptotic molecules but no change was found in caspase 9 in Neu2-overexpressed MIAPaCa2 cells compared to mock. GAPDH was used as loading control. The image was visualized and photographed. (B,C) Real-time PCR analysis of Bax, caspase3 and caspase 9 mRNA expressions in PDAC cells after Neu2-overexpression relative to mock. Values are normalized against 18S rRNA expression (n = 3 experiments).

Western blot analysis also showed higher level of Bax in Neu2-transfected MIAPaCa2 (~6.5 fold) and AsPC1 (~1.5 fold), whereas caspase 9 remained unchanged, which is a hallmark protein for the intrinsic apoptotic pathway (Fig. 2.8).

Consistent with these data, Neu2-transfected MIAPaCa2 and AsPC1 exhibited decreased level of anti-apoptotic proteins, Bcl-2 (~15.08 and 2.0 fold) respectively. PARP, a DNA-repairing enzyme also reduced in the Neu2-transfected cells compared to Mock. Overall, the reduction of Bcl-2 and up-regulation of Bax supports the notion of involvement of enhanced Neu2 in the apoptosis-regulating pathways in these transfected cells.

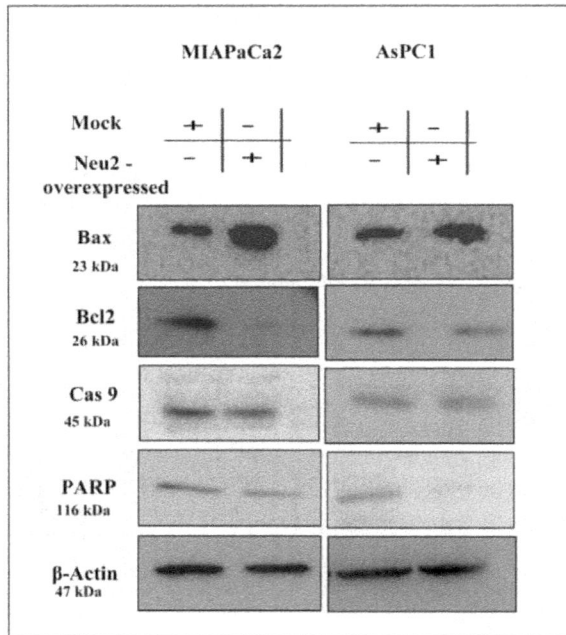

Figure 2.8 Representative immunoblots showing increased Bax, reduced level of both Bcl2 and PARP in Neu2-overexpressed PDAC cells whereas no such change was found in protein level of caspase-9. β-actin was used as loading control.

Neu2 induces reduced cell proliferation through extrinsic apoptotic pathway

Interestingly, we observed a significant increase of activated caspase 6 and caspase 8 which are hallmark proteins for extrinsic apoptosis pathway in Neu2-overexpressed MIAPaCa2 and

AsPC1 (Fig. 2.9). The cross-talk between the cell surface-mediated apoptotic signal and the mitochondria is caused by Bid hence its activation is very important. We observed cleavage of Bid along with the enhanced level of FADD. Taken together, these results suggest that caspase-8 and FADD activation along with cleaved Bid in Neu2-transfected PDAC may be induced by activation of the death receptor-mediated apoptosis.

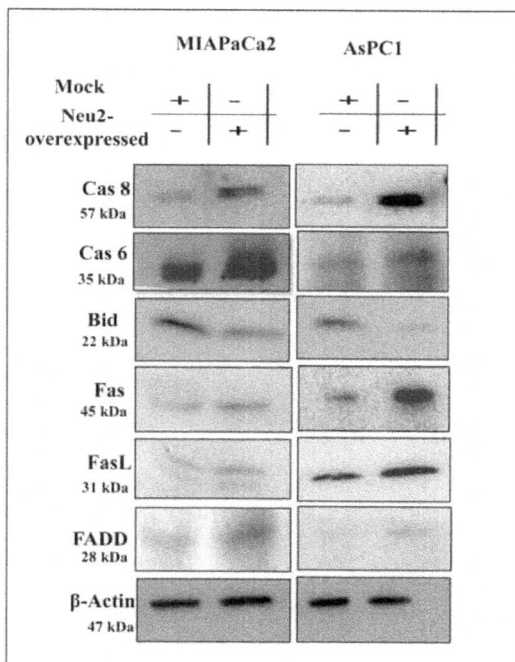

Figure 2.9 Neu2 induces apoptosis through the extrinsic-mediated apoptotic pathway. Representative immunoblots of Neu2-overexpressed MIAPaCa2 and AsPC1 cells confirmed the reduction of the protein level of Bid and enhanced caspase 8, caspase 6, Fas, FasL, FADD which are hallmark proteins of the extrinsic apoptotic pathway. β-actin was used as loading control.

Enhanced expression of Fas and FasL in Neu2-transfected cells

Next, we searched for the death receptor mechanism in Neu2-transfected cells. We observed a 1.4 and 1.6 fold upregulation of Fas/CD95 in Neu2-transfected MIAPaCa2 (Fig. 2.10A) and AsPC1 (Fig. 2.10B) respectively after 24h by flow cytometry.

Western blot analysis also suggested a significantly enhanced level of Fas and its ligand (FasL) in the transfected cells (Fig. 2.9). Therefore, it may be envisioned that though Neu2 is a cytosolic enzyme still it can stimulate apoptosis by the extrinsic pathway involving membrane bound Fas.

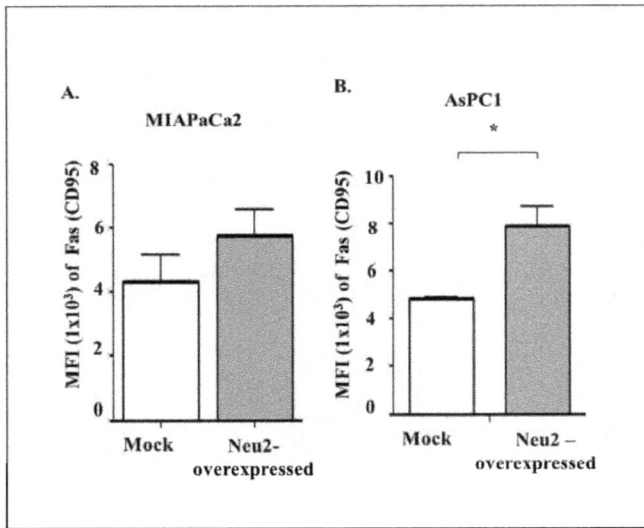

Figure 2.10 (A,B) MIAPaCa2 and AsPC1 cells were transfected with mock and PcDNA3.1-Neu2 expression vector then cells were harvested and incubated with PE-Fas (CD95) antibody for analysis by flow cytometry. Neu2-overexpressed in PDAC cells showed upregulation of Fas. The data are the means ± S.D. of three different experiments.

Neu2 reduces linkage-specific sialylation on cell surface

So far we have demonstrated presence of Neu2 on plasma membrane (Fig. 2.3B,D); accordingly, we checked whether it can reduce linkage-specific sialylation of the cell surface molecules in Neu2-transfected MIAPaCa2 (Fig. 2.10C) and AsPC1 (Fig. 2.10D) by flow cytometry. We have found reduced FITC-SNA binding with Neu2-overexpressed cells compared to mock as indicated by lower MFI value being 467.9 ± 142 vs. 607.8 ± 144.6 in MIAPaCa2 and 228.7 ± 32.68 vs. 346.7 ± 34.48 in AsPC1 respectively. In contrast, no detectable change was found when $\alpha2,3$-linked SA binding lectin (MALII) was used under similar condition (data not shown). This indicates that Neu2 possibly cleaves more $\alpha2,6$-linked sialic acids from sialoglycoproteins on the cell surface of MIAPaCa2 and AsPC1 as $\alpha2,6$-linked sialic acids is reported to be the specific substrate for Neu2.

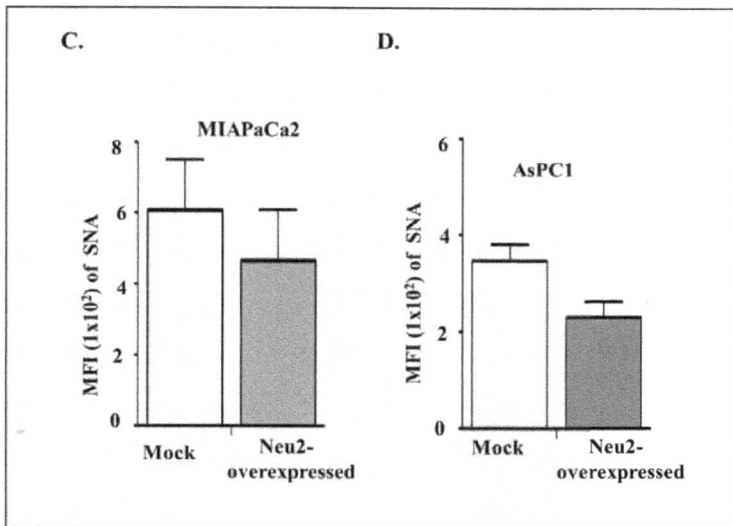

Figure 2.10 (C-D) Neu2-transfected MIAPaCa2 and AsPC1 cells exhibited decreased $\alpha2,6$-linked sialic acids. Status of sialic acids on the cell surface was demonstrated through the binding of FITC conjugated two sialic acid binding lectins (SNA and MALII). Mock and Neu2 transfected (1×10^5) MIAPaCa2 and AsPC1 cells were washed and resuspended in lectin binding buffer. Cells were incubated separately with FITC conjugated SNA for 1h. FITC positivity was acquired by FACS. Data are represented as mean $\pm$ S.D from three independent experiments

Plausible association of Neu2 on plasma membrane

As we have observed that Neu2 being a cytosolic-enzyme can induce apoptosis by the extrinsic-mediated apoptotic pathway involving Fas, so we monitored whether Neu2 is also present on the membrane. Earlier we have an indication of slightly higher enzyme activity on the membrane of Neu2-transfected MIAPaCa2 (Fig. 2.3B) and AsPC1 (Fig. 2.3D) along with less sialylation (Fig.2.10C-D).

Now the membrane fractions of these cells were immunoblotted with an anti-Neu2 antibody. We found that higher expression of Neu2 in the membrane of the Neu2-overexpressed MIAPaCa2 (Fig. 2.11A) and AsPC1 (Fig. 2.11B). E-cadherin was used to show the purification of membrane fraction. Hence, it may be stated that Neu2 is available on the membrane by an unknown mechanism.

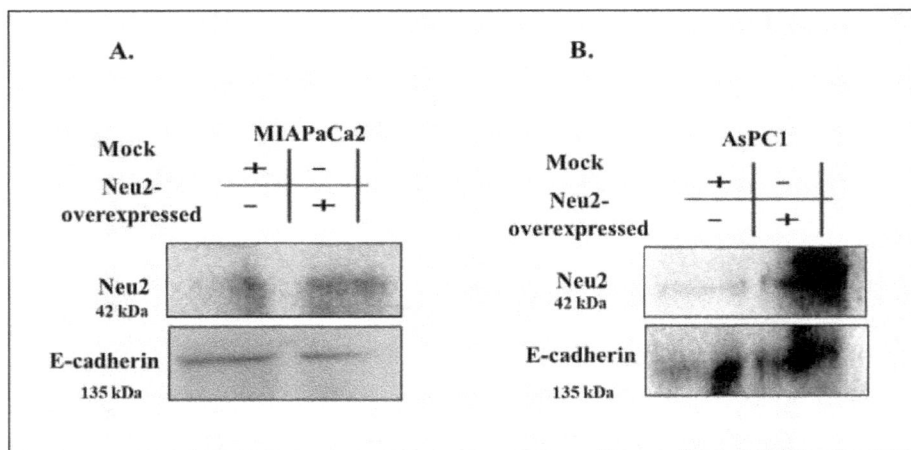

Figure 2.11 (A,B) Elevated level of Neu2 expression in membrane fraction in Neu2-overexpressed MIAPaCa2 and AsPC1 cells. Cell lysates were prepared from Neu2-transfected cells; membrane fraction was isolated by ultracentrifugation. Representative immunoblots experiment confirmed increased Neu2 expression in membrane fraction of transfected PDAC cells than mock. E-cadherin was used to show the purity of membrane preparation and also used as loading control.

Neu2 is associated with Fas death receptor

So far we have established the involvement of Fas in mediating apoptosis in Neu2-overexpressed cells through extrinsic-pathway. Now, we addressed an obvious question what is the relation between membrane-bound Neu2 and Fas. A co-immunoprecipitation with cell lysate (Fig. 2.12A) and membrane fractions (Fig. 2.12B) of Neu2-overexpressed MIAPaCa2 and AsPC1 showed that Neu2 is associated with Fas. Higher expression of membrane-bound Neu2 showed more association with the death receptor suggesting possible enhanced desialylation of Fas.

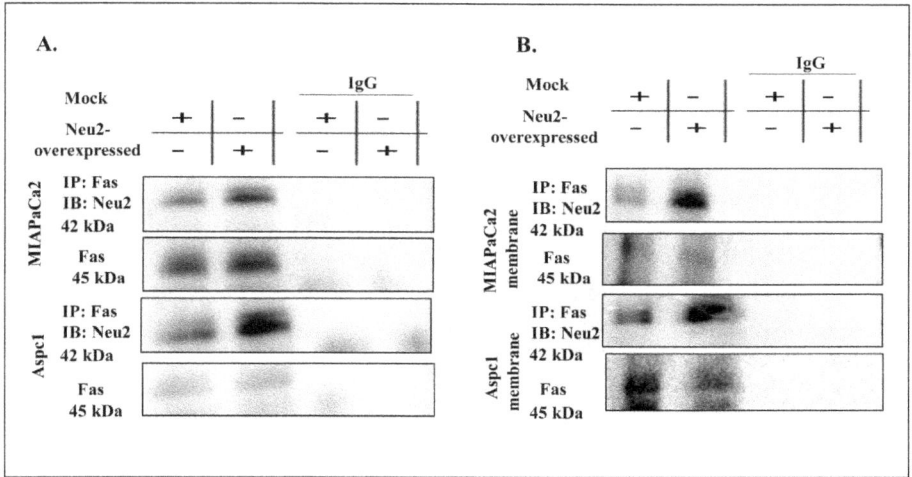

Figure 2.12 (A) Cell lysate exhibited enhanced association of Fas with Neu2 in Neu2-overexpressed cells. (B) Enhanced association of membrane-bound Neu2 with Fas in Neu2-overexpressed cells. Representative immunoblots of co-immunoprecipitation experiments of cell lysate and membrane fractions in PDAC confirmed increased binding of Fas with Neu2 in Neu2-overexpressed cells. IgG was used as negative control.

Neu2 causes desialylation of α2,6-linked sialic acids on Fas

Fas is known to have α2,6-linked sialic acids. Therefore, we checked if the Fas is the direct target for desialylation of α2,6-linked sialic acids by Neu2. A co-immunoprecipitation with cell lysate of Neu2-overexpressed MIAPaCa2 (Fig. 2.13A) and AsPC1 (Fig. 2.13B) with anti-Fas antibody and detected by SNA exhibited decreased α2,6-linked sialic acids on Fas. The band corresponding to Fas was less intense indicating that Neu2-overexpression causes its desialylation. This showed that α2,6-linked sialic acids are also present on Fas in PDAC and further reconfirms that they are the true substrate for Neu2.

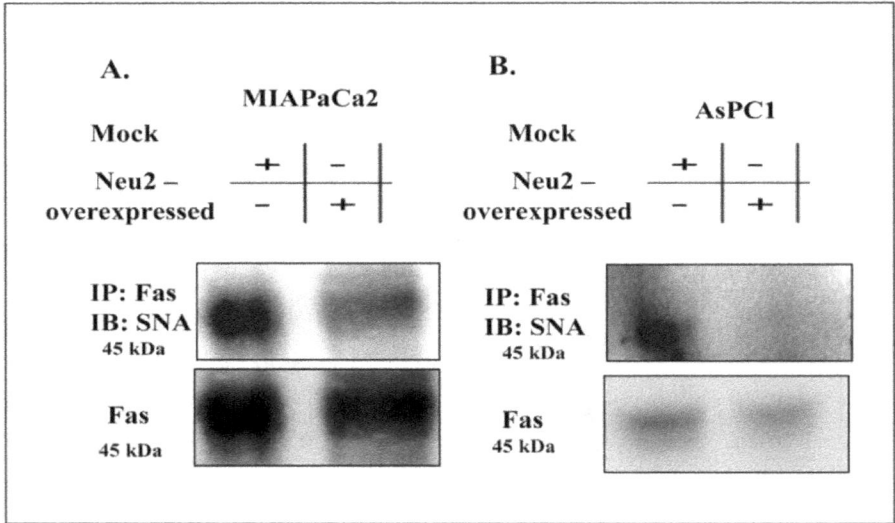

Figure 2.13 (A,B) Decreased sialylation of Fas in Neu2-transfected cells. Cell lysate from mock and Neu2-overexpressed MIAPaCa2 and AsPC1 cells were incubated with anti-Fas antibody for overnight and immunoprecipitated. Immuno-complex was resolved, and subsequently incubated with biotinylated-α2,6-linked sialic acid binding lectin (SNA) then developed by avidin-HRP antibody and detected by ECL. Lectin affinity study of Neu2-transfected MIAPaCa2 and AsPC1 cells confirmed decreased association of Fas with SNA.

2.5 Discussion

Aberrant sialylation in signalling pathways are involved in altering their functions leads to abnormal cellular-signalling causing major changes in cellular-behaviour to induce resistance to apoptosis and invasiveness.[45] Sialyltransferases and sialidases are two important players in this event. The key achievement of our study is to provide evidence for the enhancement of cytosolic Neu2 on the membrane in the Neu2-overexpressed PDAC cells. We have demonstrated for the first time a close-association of membrane-bound Neu2 with sialylated-Fas, which plays a major regulatory upstream molecule for the activation of Fas through desialylation. Activated Fas, after desialylation, enhanced several apoptotic molecules through extrinsic-apoptotic pathway caused by increased sialidase Neu2 on the membrane. Several reports suggested that higher sialylation status causes cell motility, adhesion and metastasis by modulating α2,3 sialyltransferase, ST3GalIII, galactosyl transferases in PDAC.[25] ST6Gal1 also plays an important role in regulating the invasiveness in a fructose-responsive manner.[24] This enzyme enhances α2,6-sialylation of Fas which confers protection against Fas-mediated apoptosis and facilitates tumour progression in colon cancer.[36] We have also shown α2,6-sialylation of Fas in PDAC. To the best of our knowledge, this is the first time report on Fas-sialylation in PDAC.

Expression of Neu2 is low or undetectable in several tumor cells generally with a high degree of malignancy[45]. Due to lack of adequate understanding of the mechanism by which Neu2 regulates tumour cell behaviour in pancreatic carcinoma, we aimed to explain the significance of Neu2 down regulation. Moreover, a significant strong association of lower expression status of Neu2 with clinicopathological characteristics in patient tissues has also been demonstrated. Accordingly, we over expressed Neu2 in drug resistance PDAC cells. Neu2-overexpression showed apoptosis susceptibility toward apoptotic stimuli such asserum deprivation which significantly reduced the proliferation rate. More importantly, this event pushed Neu2-overexpressed cells toward apoptosis as revealed by an increased number of cells in the late apoptotic stage by affecting important cell cycle regulatory-molecules along with increasing the expression of the pro-apoptotic and decreasing the anti-apoptotic proteins. Interestingly, caspase 6 and 8 were activated but not caspase 9 hinting for activation of the extrinsic pathway. Furthermore, we observed higher enzyme activity in the membrane fraction. This outcome gave us first notion that Neu2 probably present in the membrane in transfected cells by an unknown mechanism which desialylated α2,6-linked sialic acids of cell surface sialoglycoproteins. All these events have been demonstrated pictorially in Fig. 2.14.

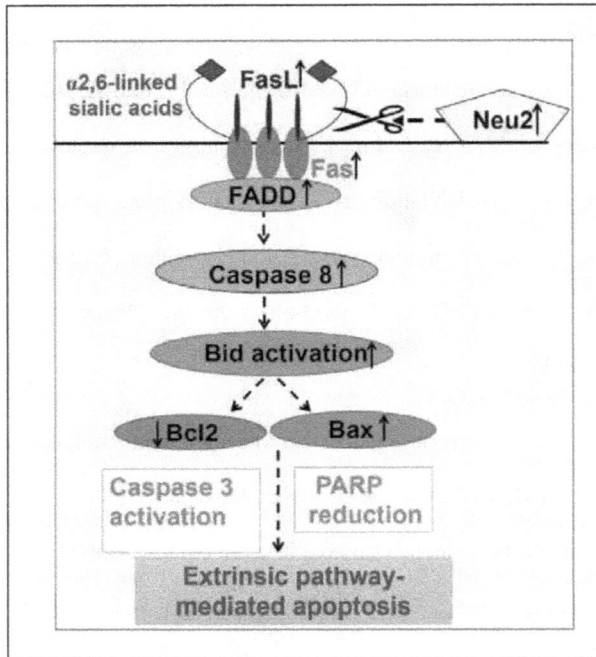

Figure 2.14 Schematic representation of Neu2-mediated regulation for desialylation of Fas and downstream signaling for inducing extrinsic-mediated apoptosis by activated Fas.

[The part of this research work has published in *Cell Death and Disease* (2018) 9:210 DOI 10.1038/s41419-017-0191-4]

CHAPTER III

Consequence of Neu2-overexpression in regulating

PI3K-AKT/mTOR signalling pathway

3.1 Aim of the study

• Differential regulation of the expression of sialoglycoproteins on cytosol due to over expression of Neu2

• Regulation of PI3K-AKT/mTOR signalling pathway after Neu2 modulation

• Deciphering the cross-talk between PI3K signalling and apoptotic pathway

• Role of transfected Neu2 on migration and invasion

3.2 Summary

This chapter covered the basic findings about the effect of Neu2-overexpression in the PI3K/Akt–mTOR signalling pathway which is known to be up-regulated in many cancers including PDAC. Neu2-overexpression in PDAC reduced the expression of several signalling molecules in this pathway. Probable desialylation of the several molecules involved in the PI3K/Akt–mTOR signalling pathway by Neu2 caused the inhibition of this pathway which in turn also causes Fas activation. Moreover, this enhanced Neu2 in PDAC cells caused decreased cell migration and invasion along with reduction in metastasis related proteins levels (VEGF, VEGFR, and MMP9). Taken together, our study establishes for the first time that Neu2 can regulate PI3K-Akt-mTOR pathway which help in the up-regulation Fas activation thus reducing cell proliferation and migration.

3.3 Introduction

PI3K–Akt pathway is upregulated in many cancers including PDAC [34,35]. Due to its constitutive activation, PDAC exhibited high metastatic potential and chemoresistance. Many of the pathway molecules are altered by sialylation[36,37]. The inhibition of PI3K–Akt pathway sometimes is responsible for the activation of Fas-mediated apoptosis in gastric, colon, and prostate cancer[38-40]. Alterations of sialylation of the PI3K pathway molecules cause inactivation of oncogenes like PI3K/mTOR resulting in regression of cancer [37]. Hence, sialidase Neu2 may play an important role in desialylation of such pathway molecules which is not fully understood. So, here in this study the effect of Neu2 on regulation of PI3K-AKT/mTOR signalling pathway have been investigated in pancreatic cancer.

3.4 Results

Neu2 mediates alterations in the sialoglycoprotein profile

To identify a possible molecular link between Neu2-overexpression and its association with Fas, we examined the status of sialoglycoproteins on membrane and cytosolic proteins of transfected cells using two plant lectins namely SNA (α2,6-sialic acid-binding lectin) and MALII lectins. (α2,3-sialic acid-binding lectin). Significant differences in SNA-binding membrane proteins were observed between Neu2-transfected MIAPaCa2 compared to mock-transfected cells (Fig. 3.1A). The major pattern changes occurred between 20 and 75 kDa proteins which underwent a marked loss of sialic acids indicating these sialoglycoproteins as the possible targets for Neu2. Ponceau S stained blot was used to indicate equal loading. Conversely, the appearance of Neu2 transfection in MIAPaCa2 caused only slight changes in the pattern of α2,3-linked sialoglycoproteins. Similar changes in the reduction of 20 and 100 kDa sialoglycoproteins profiles were observed in cytosolic proteins of transfected MIAPaCa2 (Fig. 3.1B). It may be noted that most of the molecules in the PI3K-signalling pathway are between 15 and 100 kDa and they are modulated by their sialylation status. Therefore, enhanced cytosolic Neu2 possibly has a direct role in regulating some signalling pathway by desialylation. Therefore, our observation may provide a possible link between Neu2 activity and alterations of growth factor-mediated signalling due to desialylation by Neu2-overexpression.

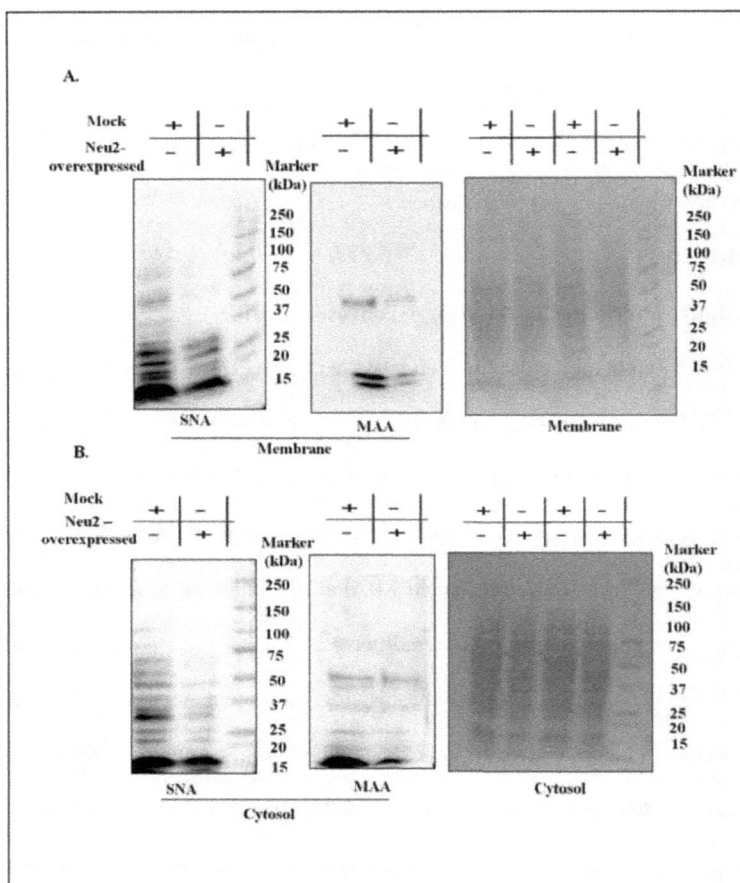

Figure 3.1 (A-B) Enhanced Neu2 modulates alterations of sialoglycoproteins in membrane and cytosolic fractions of MIAPaCa2 cells. Status of sialoglycoproteins profiles present in the membrane and cytosolic fractions purified from mock and Neu2-overexpressed MIAPaCa2 cells were assessed by lectin blotting employing both α2,6- and α2,3-linked sialic acid binding lectins namely SNA and MALII. Ponceau S stained blot was used to indicate equal loading

Neu2 impairs the activity of several signalling molecules involved in PI3K–Akt/mTOR pathway

PI3K is known to play a key role in Akt–mTOR signalling and help cancer cells to survive. Previously, we have demonstrated the association of α2,6-linked sialylated Fas with membrane-bound Neu2 and its activation through desialylation (Fig. 2.13A,B). Additionally, enhanced cytosolic Neu2 may have a direct effect on regulating PI3K pathway probably by modulation of sialylation of several molecules involved in this pathway. Inhibition of PI3K pathway causes upregulation of Fas which had earlier been reported in gastric carcinoma[38]. However, cross talk between enhanced Neu2, inhibition of the PI3K pathway and Fas activation has not been explored. Therefore, we turned our attention to the upstream proteins of this pathway involved in uncontrolled proliferation of PDAC. We observed a decreased level of PI3K in Neu2-transfected MIAPaCa2 and AsPC1 (Fig. 3.2). Neu2 overexpression inhibited PDK1 phosphorylation at Ser241. Thus this sialidase possibly reduces the PDK1-mediated Akt/mTOR signalling. PDK1 partially activates Akt phosphorylation at Thr308, we have also found decreased phosphorylation in Neu2-overexpressed cells. Furthermore, to check the effect in the intracellular phases of signalling, we evaluated specific phosphorylation level of mTOR complexes and its downstream signalling proteins in Neu2-transfected MIAPaCa2 and AsPC1(Fig. 3.3). They exhibited reduced phosphorylation at Ser2481 indicating mTORC2-specific phosphorylation. We examined the phosphorylation status of AKT at Ser473, which is a selective substrate of mTORC2 for confirming this upstream inhibition of mTORC2 signalling in these Neu2-transfected cells. We observed reduced expression of which in turn decreased the phosphorylation of its substrate AKT at the Ser473. We also detected slightly reduced levels of phosphorylation of active mTORC1 at Ser 2448 in Neu2-transfected MIAPaCa2 and AsPC1 (Fig. 3.3). As PDK1 pathway regulates mTORC1 activity which consequently controls the downstream signalling molecules, therefore, we studied the phosphorylation of S6K1 and 4E-BP1. We observed reduced phosphorylation of S6K1 at Thr389, 4EBP1 at Thr37/46, and GSK3β after overexpression of Neu2 in these cells suggesting the involvement of mTORC1 also. Taken together, all these observations suggest that overexpression of Neu2 causes reduction of growth factor-mediated several signalling molecules in the PI3K pathway, as a whole through modulation of sialylation which also could activate Fas. Thus, the activated Fas (discussed in Chapter II) possibly deregulates the overall pathways for cell proliferation and thereby forcing these cancer cells towards apoptosis.

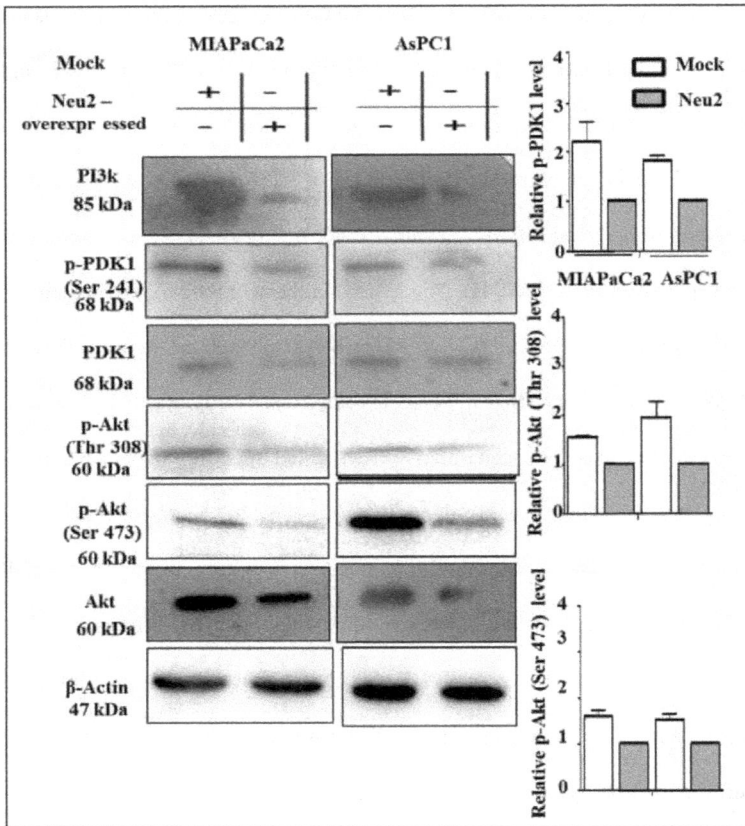

Figure 3.2 The cell lysate was prepared from mock and Neu2-overexpressed MIAPaCa2 and AsPC1 cells and resolved by SDS-PAGE, and then analyzed by western blot with the specified antibodies. Representative immunoblots showed reduction of PI3K–mTOR pathway proteins and its downstream molecules upon Neu2 overexpression in PDAC cells.

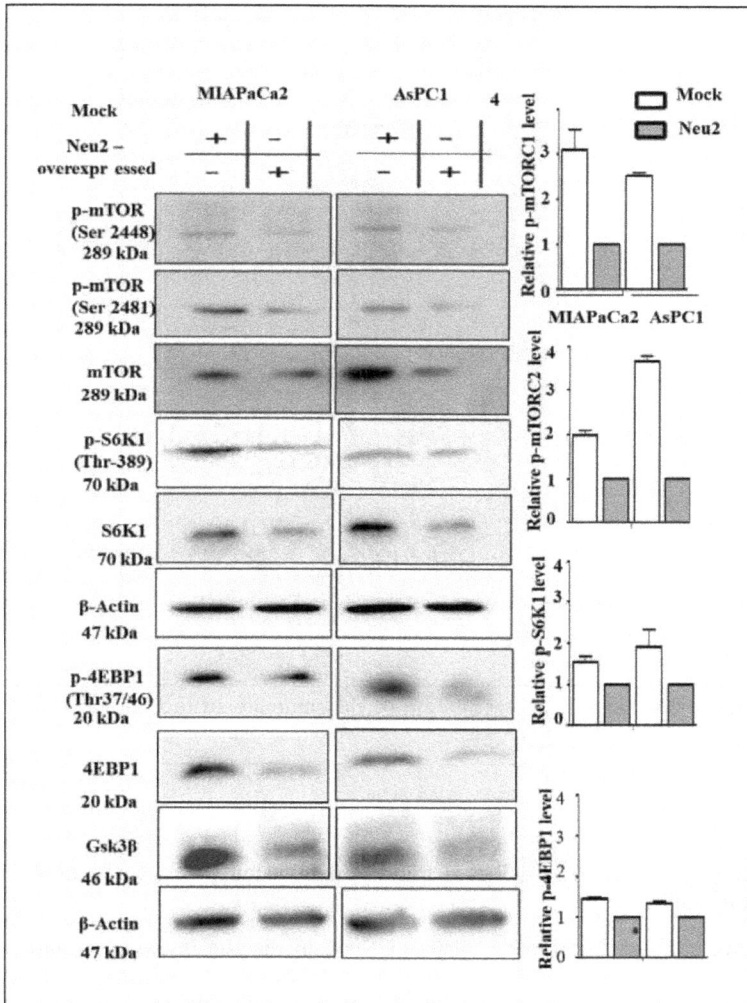

Figure 3.3 The cell lysate was prepared from mock and Neu2-overexpressed MIAPaCa2 and AsPC1 cells and resolved by SDS-PAGE, and then analyzed by western blot with the specifified antibodies. Representative immunoblots showed reduction of PI3K–mTOR pathway proteins and its downstream molecules upon Neu2 overexpression in PDAC cells.

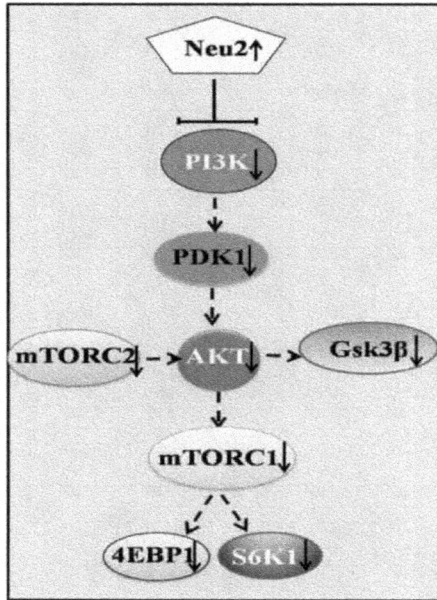

Figure 3.4 Pictorial representation of the summary of this pathway modulated by Neu2 overexpression in PDAC cells.

Enhanced Neu2 reduces cell migration and invasion through the modulation of VEGF, VEGFR, and MMP9

Next, we checked the role of enhanced Neu2 in metastasis through migration and invasion assays. We observed there was no significant change in cell migration of Neu2-overexpressed MIAPaCa2 (Fig. 3.5A-B) and AsPC1 (Fig 3.5C-D) after 8 h by scratch wound assay (Table 3.1) compared to mock.

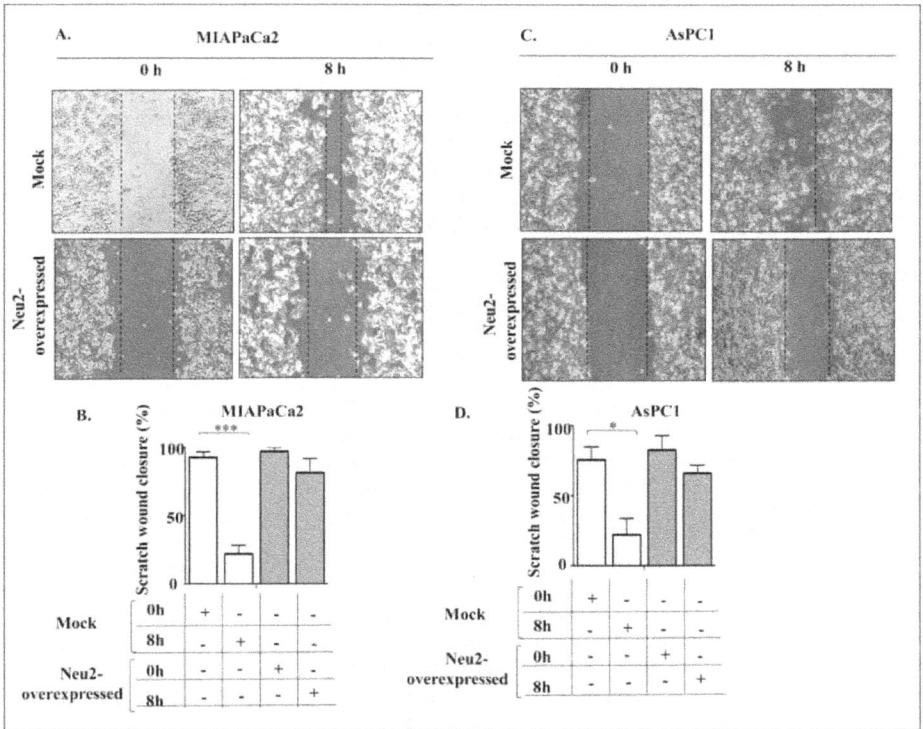

Figure 3.5 (A-D)   Inhibition of migration in Neu2-transfected MIAPaCa2 and AsPC1 cells. a MIAPaCa2 cells were transfected with mock and Neu2 plasmid in a six-well plate. In every well, a scratch was made by 2.5 µl tips. Representing images showed the filling of gaps in each well after 8 h in mock cells compared to Neu2- transfected cells. (B) Area of closure was calculated and graphically represented. (C)AsPC1 cells were transfected and processed similarly. Representing images showed minimal filling of gaps in each well in transfected cells. d Area of closures was shown. Data are represented as mean ± S.D. from three independent experiments

Additionally, we investigated the potential ability for invasiveness of Neu2-overexpressed cells. Mock-transfected MIAPaCa2 and AsPC1 invade Matrigel layer after 24 h (Fig. 3.6A). However, not much invasion of Neu2-transfected cells was observed. The number of invaded cells per-field in mock was much higher than Neu2-transfected cells (Fig. 3.6B). Taken together, Neu2-transfected cells possess less invasive property (Table 3.1).

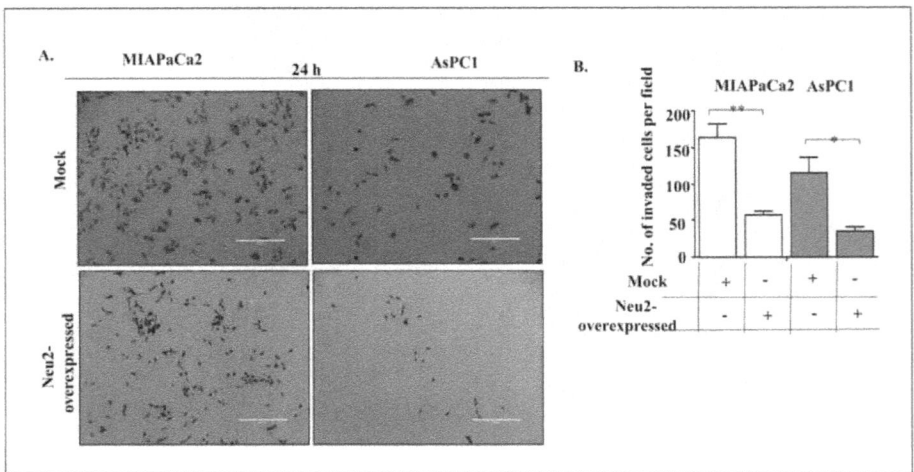

Figure 3.6 (A) MIAPaCa2 and AsPC1 cells exhibited lower invasiveness when Neu2 was overexpressed. Inverted light microscopic images of these cells showed decreased invasiveness due to Neu2 transfection. Mock-transfected cells were used as control. (B) Three randomly selected fields were counted represented graphically. Data are represented as mean ± S.D. from three independent experiments.

Table 3.1 Values of migration and invasion assay in PDAC cells

Migration assay	MIAPaCa2		AsPC1	
	Scratch wound closure (%)			
	0h	8h	0h	8h
Mock	93.30 ± 3.9	22.22 ± 5.9	75.92 ± 9.26	22.17 ± 11.5
Neu2	97.77 ± 2	82.22 ± 9.7	83.32 ± 9.62	66.57 ± 5.56
Invasion assay	: Number of invaded cells per field			
Mock	24 h		24 h	
Neu2	163.7 ± 18.35		116.0 ± 20.74	
	57.0 ± 5.13		34.67 ± 5.55	

To further strengthen the reduced inability of Neu2-transfected cells in metastasis and invasion, we have checked the status of a few specific hallmark proteins like vascular endothelial growth factor (VEGF), vascular endothelial growth factor receptor proteins (VEGFR), and matrix metalloproteinase 9 (Fig. 3.7). All these molecules were decreased compared to mock-transfected cells. Hence, it seems that not only enhanced Neu2 induces apoptosis but it can also have the potential to reduce the metastasis even in drug-resistant MIAPaCa2.

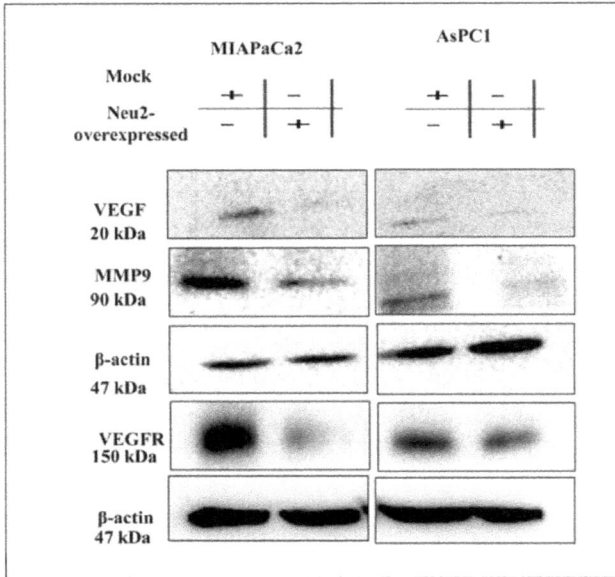

Figure 3.7 Neu2- overexpressed MIAPaCa2 and AsPC1 cells exhibited decreased level of VEGF, VEGFR, and MMP9. Representative immunoblots showed decreased proteins level of metastasis and invasiveness related proteins (VEGF, VEGFR, and MMP9) in Neu2-overexpressed PDAC cells. β-actin was used as loading control.

3.5 Discussion

Conformation changes of glycoproteins, recognition of functional molecules especially in relation to cancer progression are usually caused by removal of sialic acids which was catalyzed by a sialidase[26]. These observations comprised the preface of our study to evaluate the effects of cytosolic-sialidase Neu2, which is present in very low amount in PDAC cells. The role of Neu2 in differentiation events is an extremely regulated process[29]. Enhanced Neu2-expression leads leukemic cells towards apoptosis[41]. However; several tumour cells generally with a high degree of malignancy are lacking this sialidase[42].

One of the signalling pathways which controls cell proliferation, motility and survival is PI3K/Akt signalling pathway. During cancer this pathway is constitutively activated which helps in uncontrolled cell proliferation, leading to metastasis[35]. Molecules involved in this pathway are sialylated during cancer progression[36,37]. The activation of the Fas-apoptotic pathway by the inhibition of the PI3K/Akt pathway was reported in colon cancer[39]. It was also found that inhibition of PI3K-pathway causes Fas activation in gastric cancer and in prostate cancer[38,40]. Neu2-overexpression caused inhibition of several molecules involved in the PI3K-pathway by enhanced cytosolic-Neu2 activity which is modulated by desialylation. The effect of all these was reflected in decreased metastasis, invasiveness, and cellular proliferation due to decreased PI3K-pathway activity through modulation of sialylation which helps in upregulation of Fas activation due to enhanced Neu2.

Thus, considerable efforts have been made for understanding the molecular crosstalk between PI3K and Fas-mediated cell death in PDAC cells. Taken together, to the best of our knowledge, this is the first evidence demonstrating sialidase-Neu2 which plays as an important molecule for establishing a cross-talk by, inhibition of PI3K-pathway and activation of Fas, for induction of extrinsic-pathway and to induce apoptosis in drug-resistant human pancreatic-cancer cells. Interestingly, α2,6-linked sialic acids are considered to be the main substrate for Neu2 in pancreatic cancer. This was corroborated by the significant differences in sialylation profile of various sialoglycoproteins both in membrane and cytosol between mock and Neu2-transfected cells suggesting desialylation may be the cause of the effects which was activated by Neu2. Changes were more prominent in cleaving α2,6-linked sialoglycoproteins.

[The part of this research work has published in *Cell Death and Disease* (2018) 9:210 DOI 10.1038/s41419-017-0191-4]

CHAPTER IV

Function of the Neu2 in targeting pancreatic cancer stem-like cells (p-CSCs) by modulating Hedgehog signalling pathway

4.1 Aim of the study

- Generation of cancer stem-like cells (CSCs) from pancreatic cancer cell lines by 3D sphere culture

- Characterization of CSCs with stem cell specific molecular markers along with morphological features

- Deciphering the sialylation status in non-stem vs. pancreatic cancer stem-like cells (P-CSCs)

- Comparison of the expressions status of sialidases in non stem vs. stem-like cancer cells

- Modulation of the sialidase and deciphering its effect in sialoglycoprotein profiles of P-CSCs

- Role of the sialidase in modulation of the hedgehog signalling pathways related to the stemness of P-CSCs

4.2 Summary

This chapter covered the major findings about the role of cytosolic sialidase-Neu2 in controlling of pancreatic stem-like cells by modulation of Hedgehog (Hh) pathway. Hypersialylation is prevalent in many cancers and cancer stem-cells (CSCs), maintained by sialyltransferases/sialidases. Here, we address the involvement of sialylation in the maintenance of stemness properties of pancreatic cancer stem-like cells (pCSCs). Accordingly, we have generated pCSCs showing higher sialylation and reduced cytosolic-sialidase (Neu2) having substrate specificity towards α2,3- and α2,6-linked sialic acids. We have observed up-regulation of several molecules in hedgehog (Hh) pathway. Patient tissues also showed higher expression of sonic hedgehog (Shh) and reduced Neu2 expression. Neu2-overexpression reduced the stemness properties in pCSCs as evidenced by decreased sphere formation, stem cell-specific markers (Oct4/Sox2/Nanog) and upregulated apoptotic molecules (Bax/Cas8/Cas7/Cas3). Moreover, Neu2-overexpression downregulated PTCH1/SHH/Sufu/Smo/Gli1/Gli2/Gli3 and targeted proteins (Snail/Slug/Cyclin D1). Furthermore, enhanced association of Neu2 with Shh causing its desialylation leading to reduced Shh-Patched1 binding and demonstrated decreased expression of hedgehog-pathway molecules. Taken together, for the first time, we have demonstrated that Shh is a sialoglycoprotein with both α2,3- and α2,6-linked sialic acids. Enhanced association of Neu2 with Shh leads to its desialylation and its inhibition of binding with Patched1 resulting decreased expression of Hh-pathway molecules.

4.3 Introduction

An uncontrolled Hedgehog (Hh) signalling pathway drives tumor progression by maintaining cancer stem cells (CSCs)[43-46]. Deregulation of mTORC2 and Hh signalling help each other in increasing stemness properties in gliobalstoma multiforme[47]. Binding of Shh with pathched1 (PTCH1) protein helps in releasing of Smo molecule which further leads to activation of transcription factor Gli thereby Hedgehog-pathway (Hh) is activated[48-50]. CSCs are a population of cancer cells having self renewal and multipotency ability[51,52]. Although α2,3- and α2,6-linked sialic acids are predominant in pancreatic cancer[13,14], so far there is no information on pancreatic cancer stem-like cells (pCSCs).

Expression of cytosolic sialidase (Neu2) is very less in pancreatic cancer[53]. So far we have reported that overexpressed-sialidase (Neu2) play a significant role in balancing the overall sialylation in PDAC and thereby modulating several biological phenomena leading to apoptosis of this cancer cell as described in chapter II and III. Neu2-overexpression in pancreatic cancer cells leads to cell death by activation of extrinsic apoptotic pathway[53],(chapter II). However, the role of Neu2 in pCSCs predominantly driven by Hh-signalling pathway has received least attention.

Initially, we generated and characterized pCSCs from MIAPaCa2 and AsPC1 cell lines having different mutation status, showing higher sialylation status and up-regulated Hh-pathway molecules. These pCSCs and in patient tissues exhibited lower Neu2 as well as higher Shh than their normal counterpart. Accordingly, we aim to establish the role of Neu2 on modulation of Hh-pathway in pCSCs. Here, we demonstrated that overexpression of Neu2 causes its enhanced binding with Shh which desialylates Shh. As a result, there was decreased association of Shh with Patched1 leading to inhibition of Hh-pathway molecules. So, here in this study the effect of Neu2 on regulation of Hh signalling pathway have been demonstrated in pancreatic cancer.

4.4 Results

Generation and characterization of pancreatic cancer stem-like cells (pCSCs) from an array of pancreatic cancer cell lines

Human pancreatic cancer cell lines namely MIAPaCa2, AsPC1, PANC1 and BxPC3 having different mutation status as described before were initially used for the generation of pCSCs in non-adherent plates in stem cell specific medium for three days (chapter II). We observed that both MIAPaCa2 and AsPC1 cells originated from primary tumor and ascites respectively showed higher spheres forming ability than other two cell lines indicating differential stemness potential among these cell lines (Fig 4.1A). Therefore, we have selected MIAPaCa2 and AsPC1 cells for further experiments. Then, we characterized those spheres for CD133 and CD44 positivity through flow cytometry. All these spheres showed higher number of CD133 and CD44 positive cells than the adherent cells (Fig 4.1B). Moreover, these spheres exhibited enhanced expression of pluripotent stem cell markers, Oct4, Sox2 and Nanog in genetic (Fig 4.1C) as well as in protein levels (Fig 4.1D) as assessed by quantitative real time PCR and western blot analysis respectively. These results indicate that spheres generated from MIAPaCa2 and AsPC1 cells possess the characteristics of pancreatic cancer stem-like cells (pCSCs).

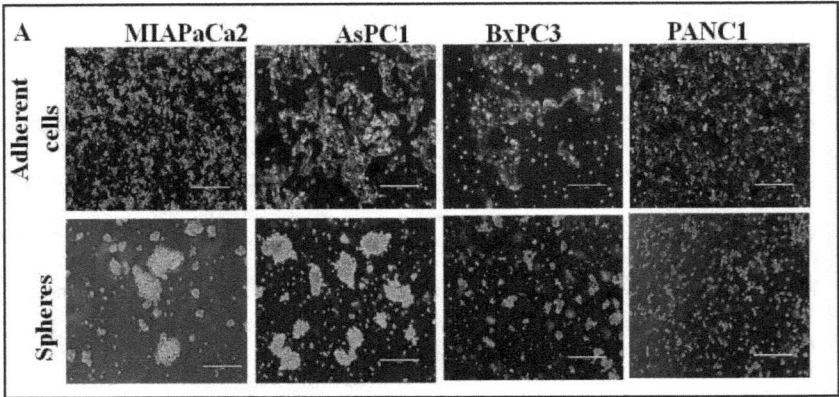

Figure 4.1 (A) Generation of pancreatic cancer stem-like cells (pCSCs) from four different human pancreatic cancer cell lines MIAPaCa2, AsPC1, PANC1 and BxPC3. Cells were cultured in non-adherent plates in stem cell specific medium containing DMEM/F12, B-27 supplements, EGF and PDGF for 3days. Representative images show differential sphere forming potential of these cells.

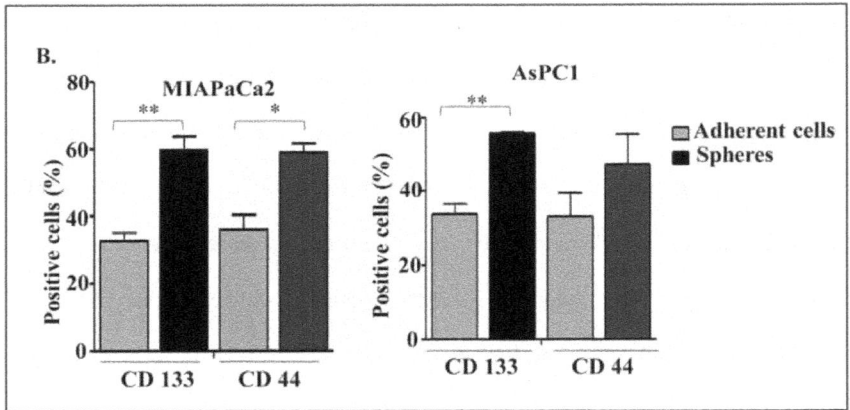

Figure 4.1 (B) Quantification of percentage of CD133 and CD44 positivity in adherent non-stem cancer and sphere cells (5 × 105) from both MIAPaCa2 and AsPC1 cells. Cells were trypsinized, washed and incubated with anti-CD133-APC and CD44-PE antibodies for 30 min at 40 C in the dark. Bar graphs were showing higher number of CD133 and CD44 positive cells in spheres.

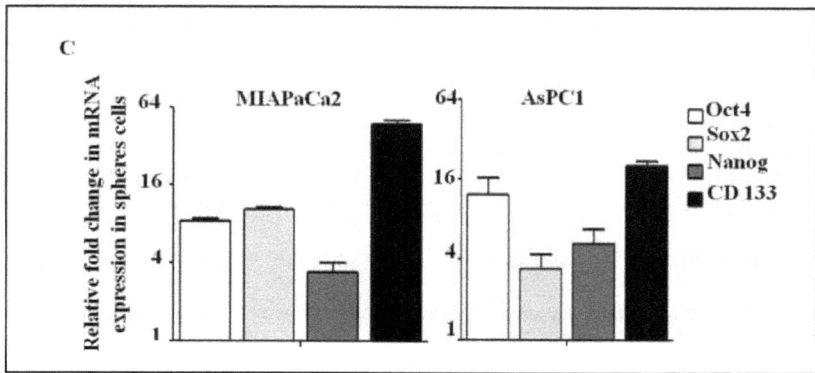

Figure 4.1 (C) qPCR analysis of adherent non-stem cancer vs. sphere cells showed higher expression of pluripotent stem cell markers such as OCT4, SOX2, NANOG and pancreatic CSCs marker CD133 in sphere cells.

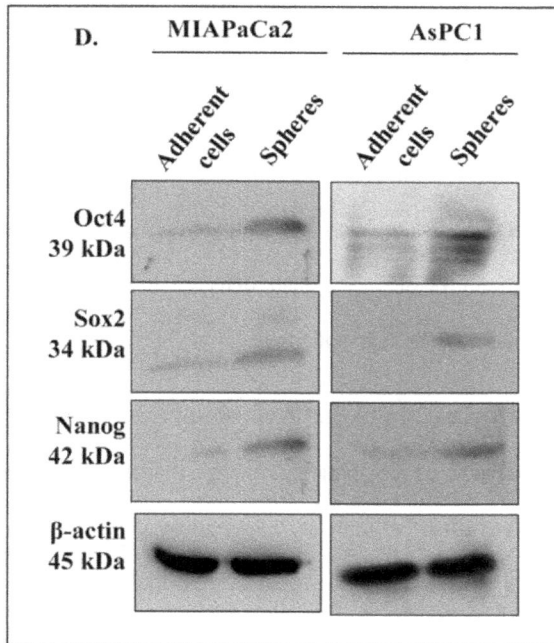

Figure 4.1 (D) Representative Immunoblots demonstrated enhanced expression of Oct4, Sox2 and Nanog at protein level in sphere cells. Adherent non-stem cancer and sphere cells were trypsinized, washed and total cell lysates were prepared and further processed for western blotting. β-actin served as a loading control.

Higher sialylation and lower sialidase (Neu2) expression in pCSCs

Next we checked the sialylation status of these pCSCs derived from MIAPaCa2 and AsPC1 cells using Sambucus nigra agglutinin (SNA) and Maackia amurensis agglutinin (MALII) lectins which binds to α2,6- and α2,3-linked sialic acids respectively (Fig 4.2A). pCSCs from both the cell lines showed a distinct higher expression of SNA-binding sialoglycoproteins than the adherent non-stem pancreatic cancer cells. However very little changes were found for MALII-binding proteins in pCSCs. Similar trends were found in surface sialylation of pCSCs detected by flow cytometry, which showed higher α2,6-linked sialylation in both the pCSCs from MIAPaCa2 and AsPC1 than the adherent non-stem counterparts (Fig 4.2B). These data indicate that pCSCs possess higher sialylation and specifically more α2,6-linked sialic acids.

One of the determinants for the expression of sialylation is sialidases, which cleaves sialic acids. So, next we checked the relative expression of sialidases in pCSCs than their adherent non-stem equivalent (Fig 4.2C). We have observed that the mRNA expression of cytosolic silaidase Neu2, which has more affinity towards α2,6-linked sialic acids, is less than other sialidases (Neu1/Neu3/Neu4) in pCSCs. We also detected higher expression of Neu1 among other sialidases which has α2,3-linkage-specificity.

We also checked the status of Neu2 in patient tissues by immunohistochemistry in randomly selected ten pancreatic cancer patient samples. Pancreatic cancer tissues showed very less expression of Neu2 than normal tissues. Optical densitometry score conferred that Neu2 expression is low in the patient tissues than their normal counterpart (Fig 4.2D).

Therefore, we can conclude that the higher expression of α2,6-linked sialic acids in pCSCs derived from both the cell lines may be due to the lower expression of sialidase Neu2 and lesser expression of α2,3-linked sialic acids may be due to higher expression of Neu1.

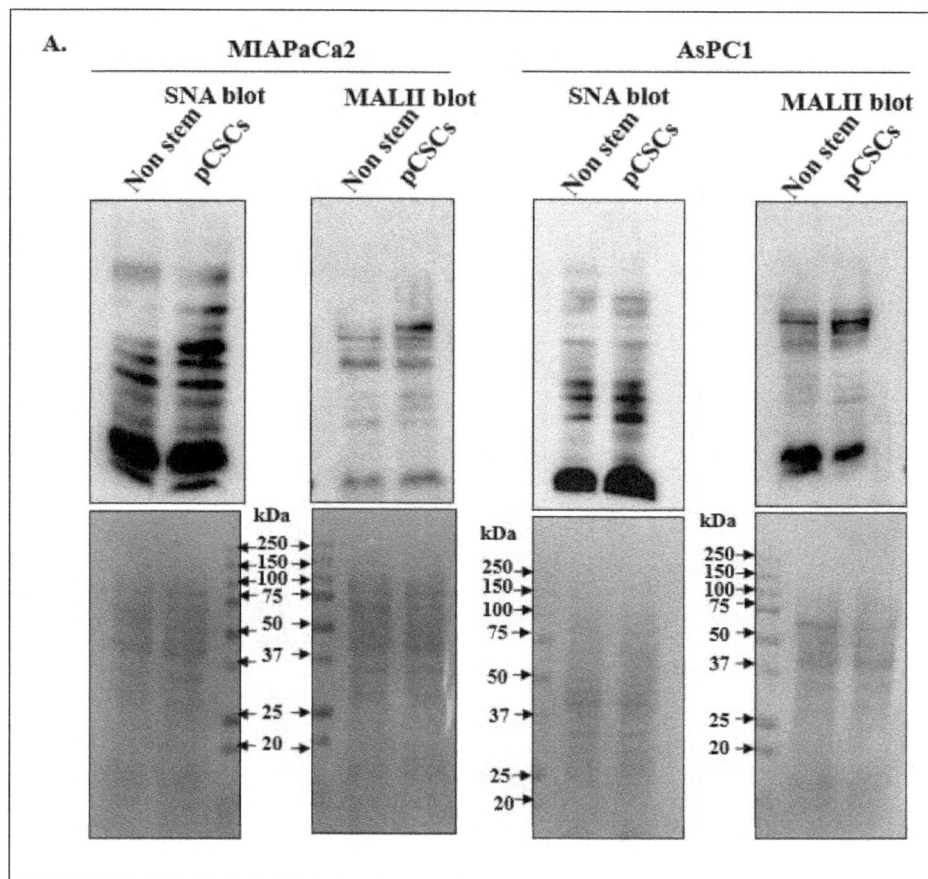

Figure 4.2 (A) Enhanced sialylation in pancreatic cancer stem-like cells (pCSCs). Cell lysates were prepared from both adherent non-stem cancer cells and pCSCs and separated electrophoretically using 10% polyacrylamide gel and further processed for western blotting. Representative blots were showing enhanced SNA and MALII binding in pancreatic cancer stem-like cells (pCSCs). PVDF membrane stained with Ponceau S used as loading control.

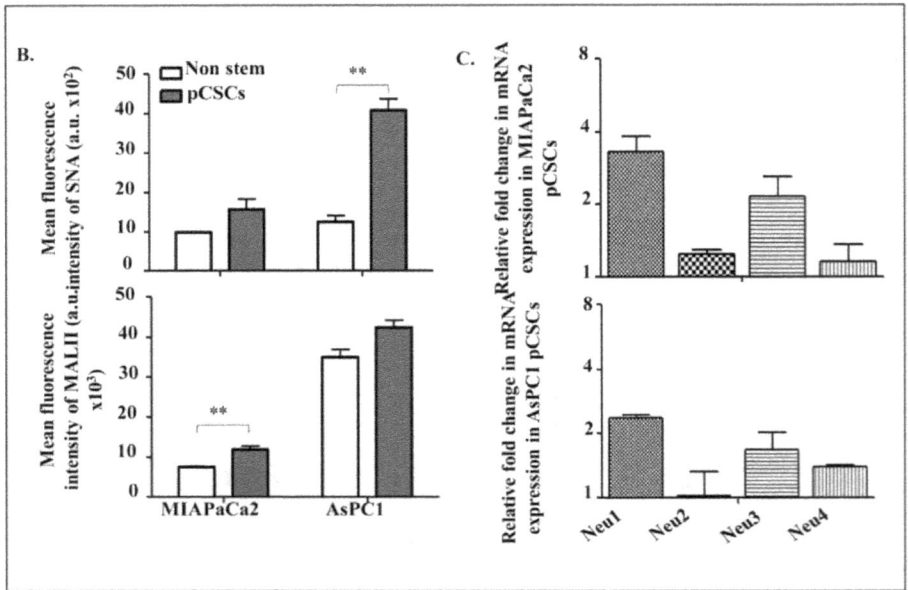

Figure 4.2 (B,C)   Enhanced sialylation and reduced sialidases in pancreatic cancer stem like cells (pCSCs).
(B) Flow cytometry analysis revealed higher surface binding of SNA and MALII with pCSCs (1 × 105) from both MIAPaCa2 and AsPC1 cells.
(C) qPCR analysis of all four sialidases namely, Neu1, Neu2, Neu3 and Neu4 in sphere vs. adherent non-stem cancer cells were determined. Relative mRNA expression of Neu2 in pCSCs compared to adherent non-stem cancer cells was lowest among other sialidases.

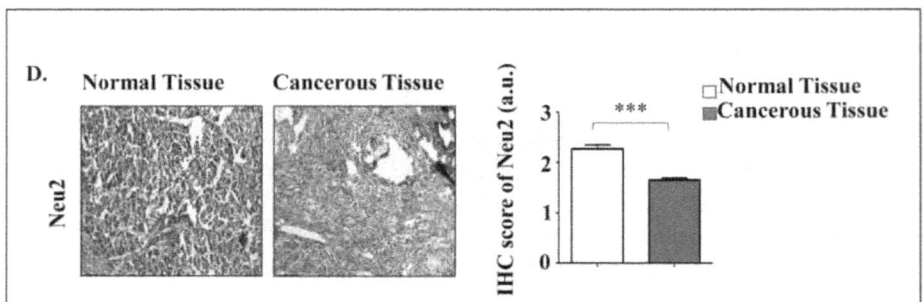

Figure 4.2 (D) Immunohistological staining showed the reduced expression of Neu2 in pancreatic tumors tissues compared to its adjacent normal tissues (20X magnification). Optical densitometry score showed significant reduction in the expression level of Neu2 in tumor tissues. Scored was measured by ImageJ software.

Neu2 over-expression reduces stemness properties in pCSCs

Further, we urged to understand whether Neu2 has any role in the maintenance of stemness in pancreatic cancers. Accordingly, we have over-expressed Neu2 in pCSCs. After 48 hrs of transfection, Neu2-overexpression was confirmed in Neu2-transfected pCSCs (NpCSCs) by western blot analysis (Fig 4.3A). Neu2-overexpression resulted in reduction of sphere-shaped morphology of these pCSCs (Fig 4.3B). NpCSCs from both the cell lines also showed lower expression of pluripotent stem cell markers such as Oct4, Sox2, Nanog both in mRNA (Fig 4.3C). and protein levels (4.3D). CD133, a known marker for pancreatic CSCs also decreased upon Neu2-overexpression in genetic level (Fig 4.3C). Corroborated with these data, the confocal images of NpCSCs also showed reduced the expression of Oct4, Sox2, and Nanog than pCSCs (Fig 4.3E). Adherent non-stem pancreatic cancer cells were used for comparison.

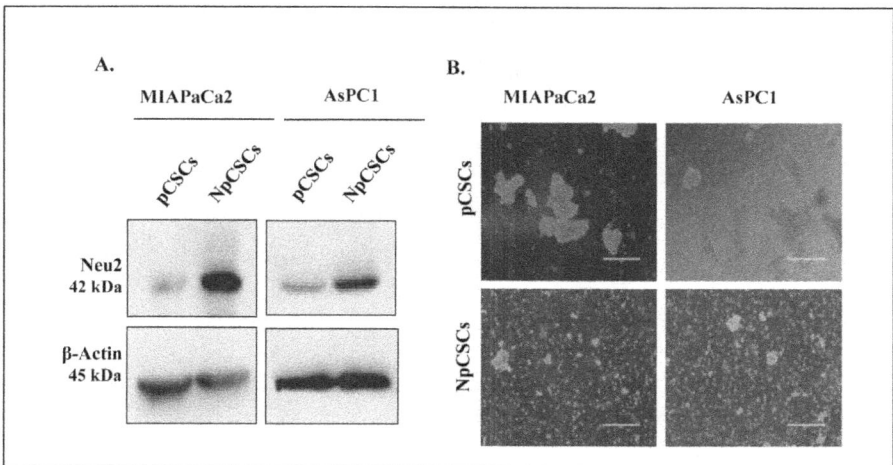

Figure 4.3 (A) Representative immunoblots exhibited higher expression of Neu2 upon overexpression in pCSCs from both MIAPaCa2 and AsPC1 cells. β- actin used as a loading control.

(B) Phase contrast images showed reduced sphere formation of Neu2-overexprssed pCSCs (NpCSCs) than pCSCs generated from both MIAPaCa2 and AsPC1 cells.

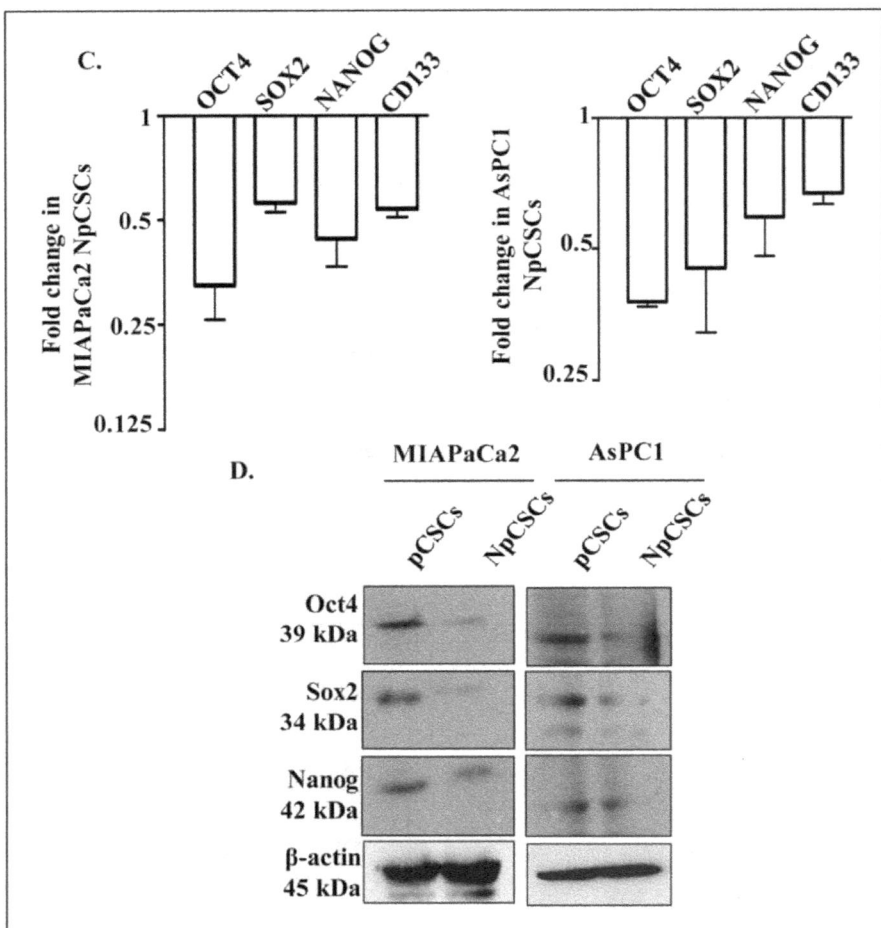

Figure 4.3 (C) Bar graph of qPCR data showed decreased expression of pluripotent stem cell markers (OCT4, SOX2, NANOG) and CD133 in NpCSCs than pCSCs from both MIAPaCa2 and AsPC1 cells.

(D) Western blot analysis demonstrated reduced expression of pluripotent stem cell markers Oct4, Sox2 and Nanog in Neu2-overexpressed pCSCs.

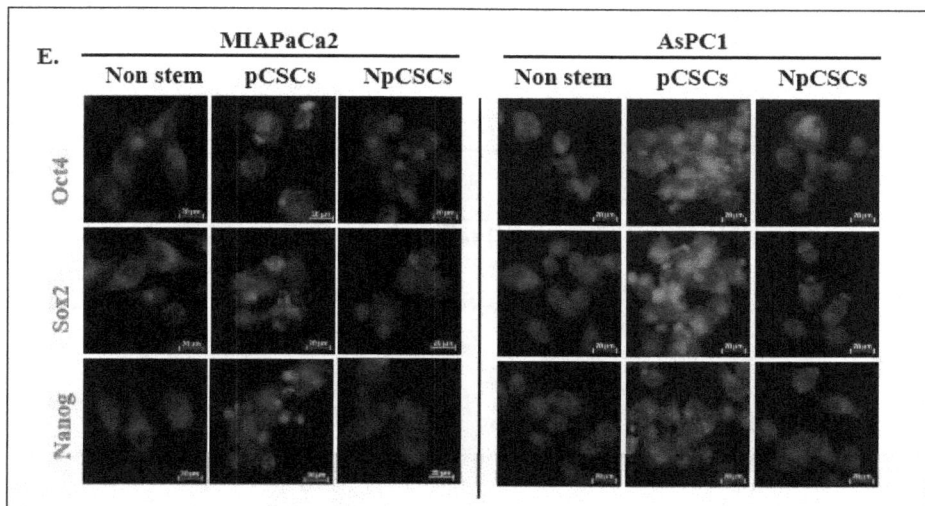

Figure 4.3 (E) Confocal microscopy images showed enhanced expression of Oct4, Sox2, Nanog in pCSCs than adherent non-stem cancer cells. Those expression were again reduced upon Neu2 overexpressed pCSCs (NpCSCs).

Reduction of sialylation and activation of apoptosis in NpCSCs

To find out whether Neu2 has any role in modulation of sialylation in pCSCs, we checked the overall sialylation status after Neu2-overexpression in pCSCs. Cell lysates from NpCSCs showed downregulation of sialylated glycoproteins as there was reduced binding with SNA and MALII than pCSCs in western blot analysis (Fig 4.4A).

Next, we compared a few apoptotic molecules between pCSCs and NpCSCs. We observed higher expression of pro-apoptotic molecules such as Caspase 3, 7, 8, and Bax and lower expression of anti-apoptotic Bcl2 in NpCSCs both in mRNA (Fig 4.4B) and protein (Fig 4.4C) levels compared to pCSCs. However no such change was found in Caspase 9, a hallmark protein for intrinsic pathway-mediated apoptosis. This was corroborated with our earlier observation wherein we have reported that Neu2-overexpression activated extrinsic pathway of apoptosis in pancreatic cancer cell lines[53.]

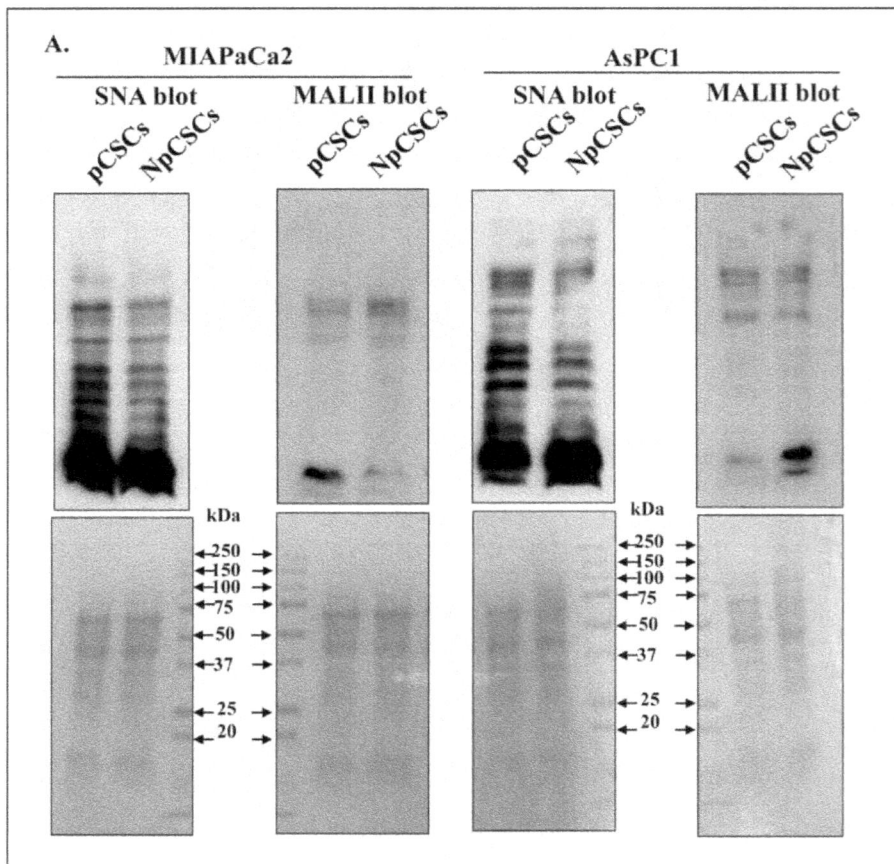

Figure 4.4 (A) Representative blots exhibited reduced SNA and MALII binding with NpCSCs compared to pCSCs. Cell lysates were prepared and electrophoretically separated using 10% polyacrylamide gel and further processed for western blotting. PVDF membrane stained with Ponceau S used as loading control.

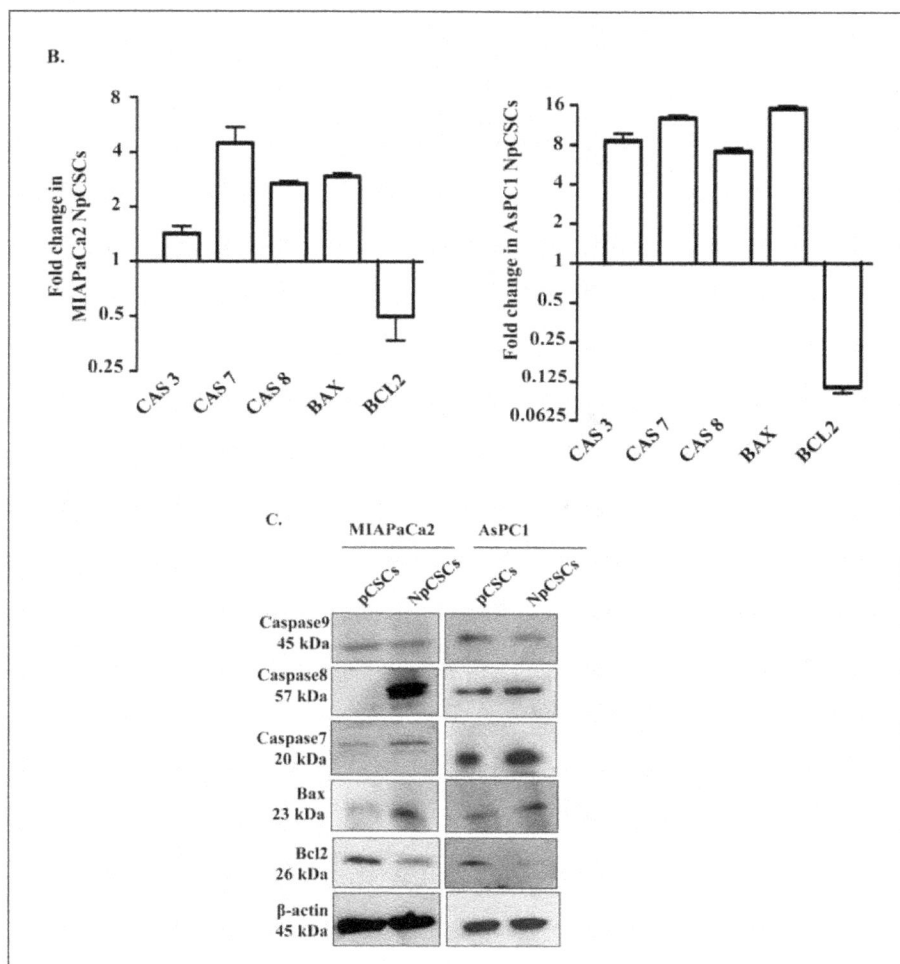

Figure 4.4 (B) qPCR analysis were showing higher expression of pro-apoptotic genes such as CAS 3, 7, 8 and BAX and reduced expression of anti apoptotic BCL2 in Neu2-overexpressed pCSCs from both MIAPaCa2 and AsPC1 cells.

(C) Western blot analysis illustrated higher expression of pro-caspase proteins such as Caspase 7, 8 and Bax along with reduced expression of Bcl2 in NpCSCs. β-actin served as a loading control.

Neu2-overexpression in pCSCs diminishes Hedgehog pathway (Hh) activity

Hh-pathway is frequently hyperactivated in cancer which regulates several genes leading to cell proliferation and helps in cancer stem cells renewal and regeneration. So, next we have checked the expression of Hh-pathway specific molecules in pCSCs generated from both the cell lines. We have found higher expression of Patched1 (PTCH1), Shh, Sufu, Smo, Gli1, Gli2 and Gli3 both in mRNA (Fig 4.5A) and protein levels than adherent non-stem cancer cells (Fig 4.5B). We have also assessed expression of Shh in patient tissues by immunohistochemistry in randomly selected ten pancreatic cancer patient samples. Representative images showed an enhancement of Shh protein in pancreatic cancer tissues suggested their aggressiveness (Fig 4.5C). Optical densitometry score conferred that higher expression of Shh found in cancer tissue than their normal counterparts. Therefore, low sialidase Neu2 expression probably help in higher sialylation in cancer and maintaining stemness as evidenced by higher Shh expression.

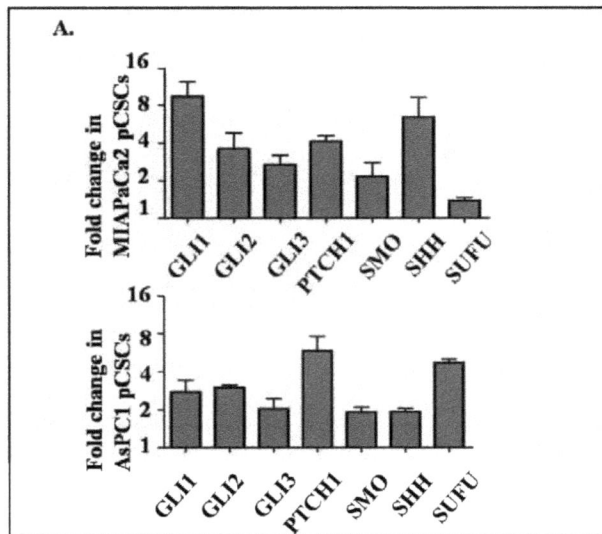

Figure 4.5 (A) qPCR data were representing enhanced expression of hedgehog pathway genes such as PTCH1, GLI1, GLI2, GLI3, SMO, SHH and SUFU in pancreatic cancer stem-like cells generated from both MIAPaCa2 and AsPC1 cells.

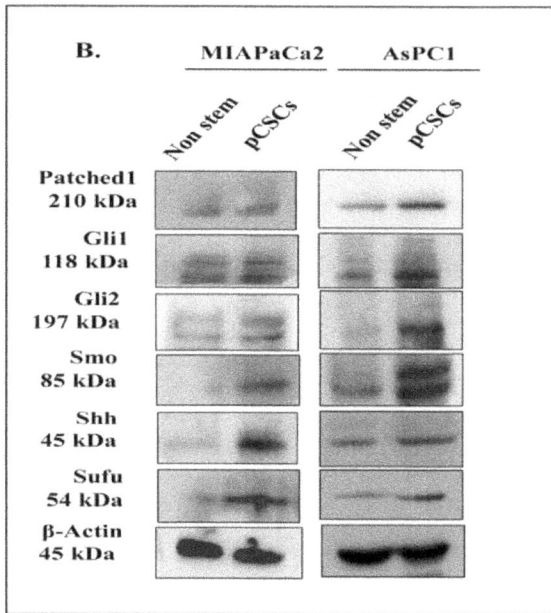

Figure 4.5 (B) Representative immunoblots exhibited higher expression of several Hedgehog pathway proteins like Patched1, Gli1, Gli2, Smo,Shhand Sufu in pCSCs than adherent non stem cancer cells in both MIAPaCa2 and AsPC1 cells. β- actin used as a loading control.

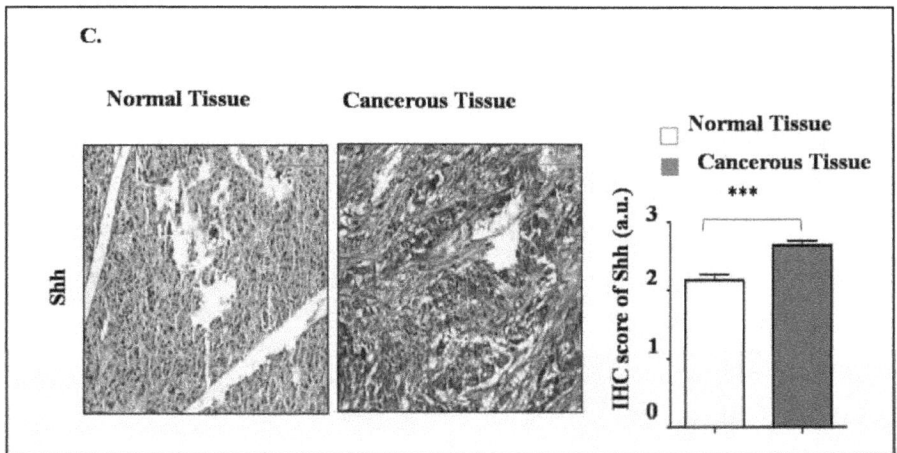

Figure 4.5 (C) Immunohistological staining of pancreatic tumors and adjacent normal tissues showed the enhanced expression of Shh in cancer tissues. The tissue samples were photographed at 20X magnification. Optical densitometry score showed significant changes in the expression level of Shh. Scored was measured using ImageJ software.

To prove our hypothesis, we checked the status of Hh-pathway molecules after Neu2-transfection in pCSCs (NpCSCs). Corroborated with our hypothesis, the expression of Pathched1 (PTCH1), Shh, Sufu, Smo, Gli1, Gli2 and Gli3 are down-regulated in NpCSCs as evidenced by lower mRNA (Fig 4.5D) and protein levels compared to pCSCs (Fig 4.5E). Therefore, we can conclude that Neu2 plays an important role in the maintenance of pCSCs by modulation of Hh-pathway.

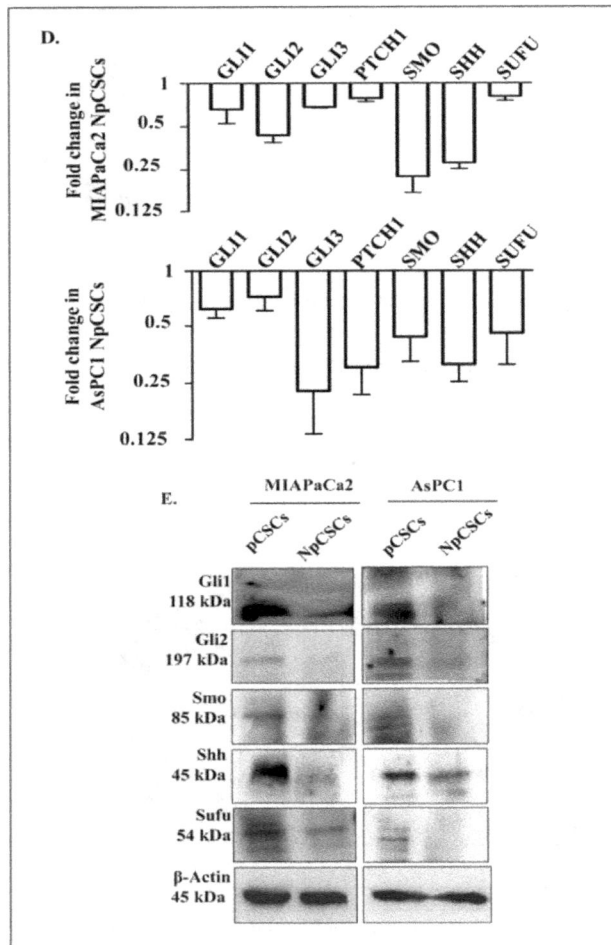

Figure legend continued on next page

Figure 4.5 (D) qPCR analysis showed reduced expression of Hedgehog pathway genes such as PTCH1, GLI1, GLI2, GLI3, SHH, SUFU, SMO in Neu2-overexpressed pCSCs generated from both MIAPaCa2 and AsPC1 cells.

(E) Representative immunoblots demonstrated decreased expression of Gli1, Gli2, Smo,Shh, andSufuin NpCSCs than pCSCs from both MIAPaCa2 and AsPC1 cells. β-actin used as loading control.

Association of Neu2 with sonic hedgehog (SHH) causes its desialylation and deactivation

So far, we have shown that overexpression of Neu2 modulates Hh-pathway in pancreatic cancer stem-like cells. Next, we wanted to address the mechanism of such modulation of Hh-pathway by Neu2. Co-immunoprecipitation of Neu2 with Shh showed higher association of Neu2 with Shh in NpCSCs generated from both the cell lines (Fig 4.6A). Furthermore, co-immunoprecipitation of Shh with SNA showed less association suggesting desialylation of highly glycosylated Shh in NpCSCs compared to pCSCs (Fig 4.6B). Similar trend was observed when Shh co-immunoprecipitated with MALII. In this experiment, for the first time, we demonstrated that Shh is a sialoglycoprotein having both α2,6- and α2,3-linked sialic acids in pCSCs.

Moreover, we have checked the association of Shh with Patched1 which facilitate the release of Smo to further activate the downstream signalling. Co-immunoprecipitation with Shh and developed with Patched1 exhibited less association of Shh with Patched1 in Neu2-overexpressed pCSCs (NpCSCs) compared to pCSCs (Fig 4.6C). Hence, it proves that association of desialylated SHH in Neu2-overexpressed condition unable to bind with Patched1 which helps in down-regulating Hh-pathway in NpCSCs.

Furthermore, Neu2-overexpression caused reduction of Hh-pathway target genes such as Cyclin D1, Slug and Snail in pCSCs due to desialylation and deactivation of Shh molecule (Fig 4.6D).

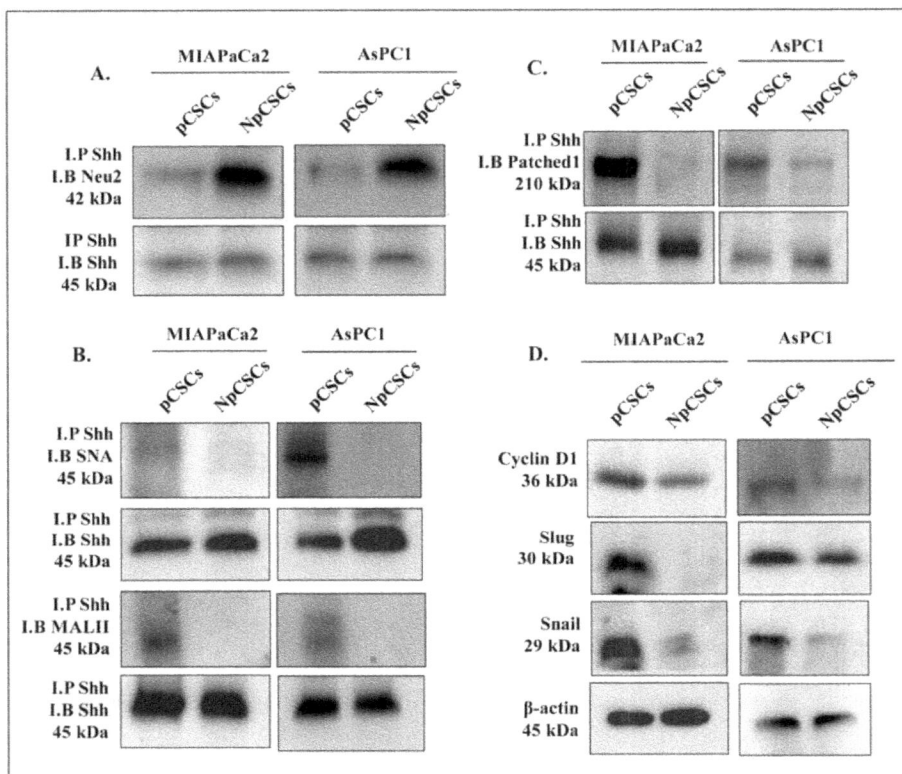

Figure 4.6 (A-D) Impaired association of Shh with Patched1 due to desialylation of Shh by overexpressed-Neu2

(A) Co-immunoprecipitation of Neu2 and Shh showed higher association in NpCSCs than pCSCs.

(B) The immuno-complexes were also identified using the SNA and MALII respectively to illustrate reduced α2,6- and α2,3-linked sialylation of Shh in NpCSCs. Immunoblots with anti-Shh antibody served as loading control.

(C) Co-immunoprecipitation showed decreased association of Patched1 and Shh in NpCSCs. This was performed as described in materials and methods. Immunocomplex was identified using the anti-Patched1 antibody. Immunoblots of Shh served as loading control.

(D) Representative western blots showed reduced expression of Hedgehog pathway target proteins such as Cyclin D1, Slug and Snail in NpCSCs. β-actin used as loading control.

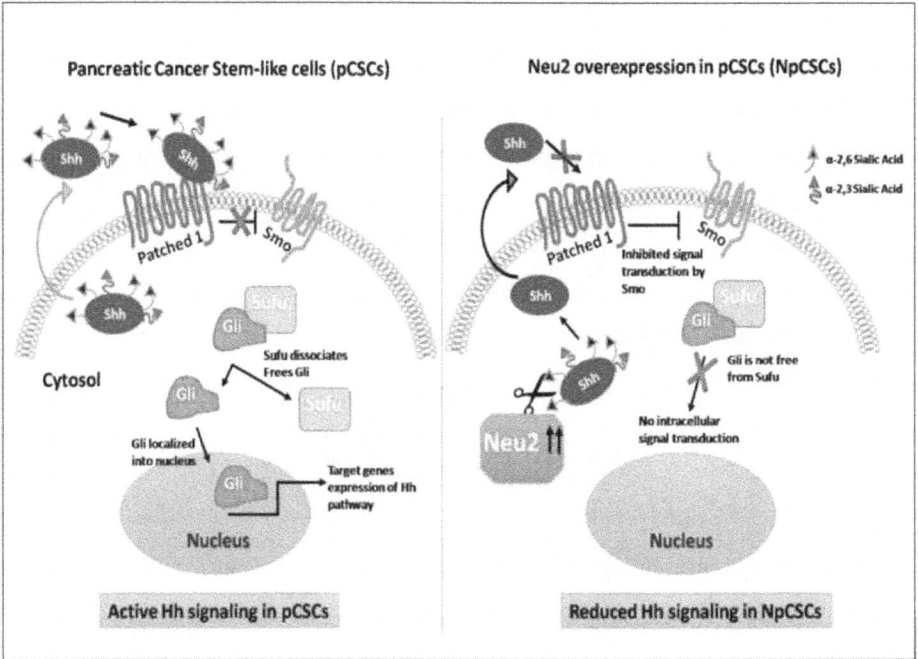

Figure 4.7 Schematic diagram highlighting reduced association of Shh with Patched1 in NpCSCs due to removal of sialic acids on Shh by overexpressed-Neu2. As a result, Hedgehog signalling cascade is downregulated by inhibiting Smo and reducing the expression of Sufu and Gli proteins.

4.5 Discussion

The drug resistant cancer cells generally possess self-renewal and differentiation properties and are considered the main source of tumorigenesis and termed as CSCs[54]. Higher sialylation is one of the key features of CSCs which is associated with tumor aggressiveness[55].

The key achievement of our study is to provide the evidence that Neu2 regulates stemness properties of pancreatic cancer cells by desialylating the important molecule in hedgehog pathway. We have demonstrated for the first time that Shh, an important molecule in Hh pathway, is a sialoglycoprotein having both α2,6- and α2,3-linked sialic acids. The association of Shh with Patched1 is the first and absolutely necessary step for the successful initiation of downstream signalling of Hh-pathway. Our data demonstrate that sialylation of Shh is important for this association with Patched1. However, Neu2-overexpressed pancreatic cancer stem-like cells (pCSCs) showed a close association of Neu2 with Shh which leads to desialylation of Shh. Desialylated Shh unable to bind with Patched1 causing deactivation of the Hh-pathway.

Due to such reduced expression of Neu2, we have described in chapter II that higher sialylation both in MIAPaCa2 and AsPC1 having K-RAS activating and p53 inactivating mutation indicating more aggressiveness of these cells[53]. Reduced expression of Neu2 was also reflected in the sphere formation capacity as well as higher sialylation status in the pCSCs generated both from MIAPaCa2 and AsPC1.

Among other three sialidases (Neu1, Neu3 and Neu4), expression of Neu2 was found to be lowest in these pCSCs which is possibly responsible for such higher sialylation specially α2,6-linked sialic acids, a substrate for this sialidase. For the detection of the significance of this sialidase in controlling the stemness property in pCSCs, we overexpressed Neu2 in these cells.

Sialylation plays an important role in regulating pluripotency and differentiation in stem cells and also involved in crucial cell fate decision[56,57]. Hence, the up-regulation of this sialidase in cancer stem-like cells which cleaves sialic acids from glycoproteins and oligosaccharides expected to deregulate the stemness property. Affirmatively, we demonstrated Neu2-overexpression caused not only reduction of the sphere shaped morphology but also several stem cell-specific molecules like Oct4, Sox2 and Nanong in these NpCSCs. Furthermore, this up-regulation of sialidase caused reduction in the sialoglycoproteins profile. Hence, this detrimental effect in the modification of the sialylation profile by Neu2-overexpression directed these NpCSCs towards apoptosis as exhibited by increase in the pro-apoptotic molecules (Bax/caspase8/caspase7/caspase3) and decrease in the anti-apoptotic molecule. This was corroborated with our earlier report that Neu2-overexpression guides up-regulation of Fas, FasL and FADD leading to activation of caspase8 and Bid cleavage thus inducing extrinsic pathway-mediated apoptosis not only in PDAC cells [53] but also in ovarian cancer cells (personal communication). Therefore, this may be hypothesized that cytosolic sialidase Neu2 in general preferentially aiming the extrinsic pathway-mediated apoptosis through targeting several membrane-bound molecules not only in different cancer cells even in cancer stem-like cells.

Hh-pathway is an important signal transduction pathway for the maintenance and proliferation of cancer stem-like cells[58]. pCSCs generated from MIAPaCa2 and AsPC1 cell lines also showed higher activation of Hh-pathway than the adherent non-stem cancer cells. Lower expression status of Neu2 and higher expression of Shh were found even in patient tissues. These observations comprised the preface of our study to evaluate the effects of Neu2 on Hh-pathway in pCSCs. Neu2-overexpression caused down-regulation in Hh signalling pathway in pCSCs. Shh is the main driving molecule for activation of this pathway[59]. We had observed enhanced association of Shh with Neu2 in NpCSCs. Such association leads to desialylation of Shh which was confirmed by reduced SNA and MALII binding suggesting presence of linkage-specific sialic acids on Shh. Although glycosylation in Shh is reported in bladder cancer[59] this is the first report for the presence of sialylated Shh in pCSCs.

Both Shh and Patched1 are upstream molecules for activation of this Hh pathway (ref). Association of Shh and Patched1 is required to release Smo molecule needed to switch on this pathway[60]. This association is drastically hindered when sialic acids were removed from Shh in NpCSCs due to Neu2-overexpression which down-regulate the Hh pathway. More importantly, this event shoved Neu2-overexpressed pCSCs toward apoptosis as revealed by modulation of the pro and anti-apoptotic molecules suggesting Neu2 as promising target for initiation of cell death in pancreatic cancer stem-like cells.

[This part of the work is currently under review in UGC approved international peer reviewed journal 'MDPI-CELLS']

CHAPTER V

Effect of inhibition of mTORC2-GSK3β axis by Neu2 over-expression regulates Hh pathway to maintain stemness of pancreatic cancer stem-like cells (p-CSCs)

5.1 Aim of the study

- Deciphering the crosstalk between Neu2 and mTORC2-Gsk3β axis in pancreatic cancer stem-like cells (P-CSCs)

- Crosstalk between Rictor on stemness of pCSCs in the context of Neu2

- Consequence of Hh pathway molecules due to modulation of Rictor and Neu2 in P-CSCs

- Role of overexpressed-Neu2 on tumour generated in NOD/SCID mice model

5.2 Summary

This chapter covered the basic findings about the effect of cytosolic sialidase-Neu2 in regulating the mTORC2-Gsk3β axis, which cross-talk with Hedgehog (Hh) pathway to retain the stemness properties of the pancreatic cancer stem-like cells (pCSCs). Neu2-overexpression showed lower mTORC2 formation and decreased hedgehog-pathway molecules by downregulating inhibitory phosphorylation of Gsk3β at serine 9 position in pCSCs. Rictor-overexpression (a main component of mTORC2) confers upregulation of stem-cell markers and hedgehog-pathway molecules. However, upon co-transfection, Neu2-overexpression reversed the effect of Rictor-overexpression. Furthermore, Neu2-overexpressed pCSCs showed reduction of tumor size and volume in NOD/SCID mice along with downregulation of stem cell markers, upregulation of apoptotic molecules, Shh and mTOR. Moreover, molecular cross-talk between mTORC2 and Hh-pathways in the context of global change in sialylation by Neu2-overexpression led to reduce stemness in pCSCs due to modulation of Hh-pathway. Deciphering such underlying mechanism of molecular interplay of sialylated Shh-Patched1 and mTORC2-Hh pathway axis through modulation of sialic acids possibly pave the way for the management of pCSCs.

5.3 Introduction

The mammalian target of rapamycin (mTOR) is up-regulated in cancer stem cells (CSCs) which increases sphere formation indicating self-renewal property of stem-like cells, thus mTOR increases stemness properties in CSCs[61,62]. Deregulation of mTORC2 (a form of mTOR which contains main molecule Rictor) and Hh signalling help each other in increasing stemness properties[47]. Additionally, mTORC2 signalling also facilitates Hh-pathway activity by inhibition of ubiquitinylation of Gli proteins through inhibitory phosphorylation of GSK3β molecule[47]. Constitutive activation of these pathways in CSCs leads to tumor cell survival[61]. Additionally, involvement of mTORC2 which sequentially control the aberrant Hh-pathway regulation in pCSCs has also not been addressed in the context of Neu2. In chapter III, we have observed reduced expression of mTORC2 upon Neu2-overexpression in pancreatic cancer cells which was caused through probable desialylation. Here, also in Neu2-overexpressed pCSCs reduced mTORC2 formation was observed which caused decreased Hh-pathway genes by down-regulating inhibitory phosphorylation of Gsk3β. However, overexpression of Rictor leads to improved stemness and higher Hh activity. Co-expression of Rictor and Neu2 reverse this phenomena indicating modulation of pCSCs characteristics both via mTORC2 signalling and SHH desialylation through Neu2. Furthermore, this was corroborated by *in vivo* study where Neu2 over-expression causes reduction of tumor size and volume in NOD/SCID mice. Moreover, we found that Neu2 over-expression in tumor tissue down-regulates stem cell markers, Shh and mTOR proteins and up-regulates pro-apoptotic genes (BAX, CAS3, CAS8). Here, we have revealed the underneath molecular cross talk between Neu2/mTORC2/Hh-pathways in pCSCs.

5.4 Results

Neu2 downregulates mTORC2 formation

Mammalian target of rapamycine (mTOR) is known to be associated with cancer progression as well as CSCs maintenance. Rictor is the essential component to form mTOR complex 2 (mTORC2) whereas Raptor is needed to form mTORC1. We have earlier reported less mTORC1 and mTORC2 levels in Neu2-overexpressed pancreatic cancer cells (chapter III).

Here, we compared the status of mTORC2 and its associated signalling pathway molecules in the pCSCs compared to adherent non-stem pancreatic cancer cells. We observed higher mTORC1/2 formation in pCSCs generated from both the cell lines as depicted by the elevated phosphorylation of mTOR both at serine 2448 and 2481 position respectively compared to adherent non-stem pancreatic cancer cells (Fig 5.1A). Further, we confirmed that these complex formations were facilitated by negative phosrylation of GSK3β at Ser 9 position and positive phosphorylation of AKT at Ser 473 position in pCSCs (Fig 5.1B). Subsequently we also compared their status between pCSCs and NpCSCs. Neu2-overexpression caused the downregulation of mTORC1/2 formation in pCSCs as evidenced by the lower phosphorylation of mTOR at serine 2448 and 2481 position and lower expression of Raptor and Rictor respectively in both the cell lines (Fig 5.2A). We also observed lower negative phosphorylation of GSK3β at Ser 9 position and reduced positive phosphorylation of AKT at Ser 473 position suggesting decreased survival of pCSCs upon Neu2-overexpression (Fig 5.2B).

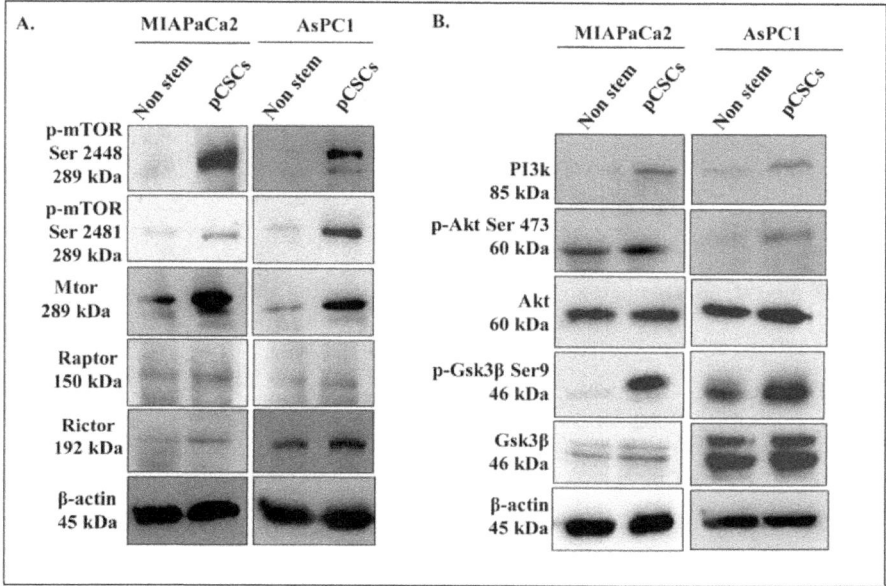

Figure 5.1 (A) Representative immunoblots exhibited enhanced mTORC1/2 formation and higher expression of Rictor and Raptor in pCSCs from both the cell lines. β-actin used as a loading control.

(B) Western blots analysis were showing inhibition of Gsk3β and activation of Akt in pCSCs from both the cell lines. β-actin used as a loading control.

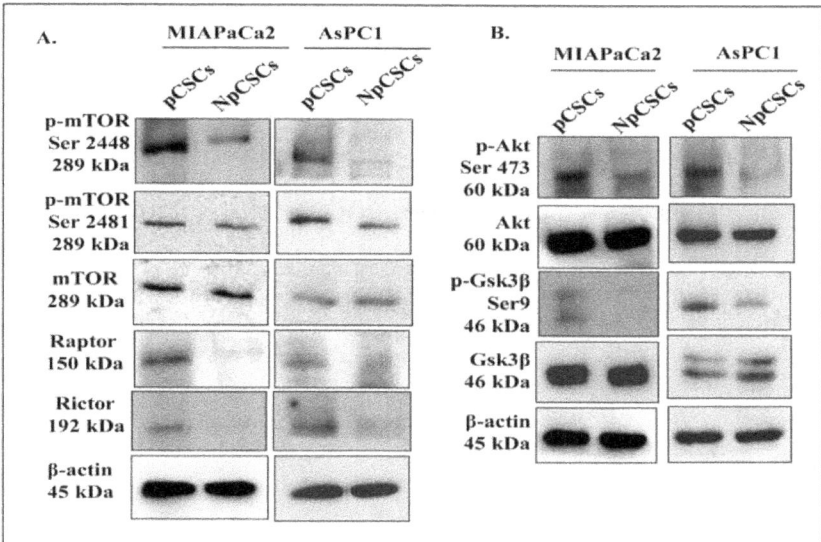

Figure legend continued on next page

Figure 5.2 (A) Representative immunoblots exhibited reduced mTORC1/2 formation and decreased expression of Raptor and Rictor in NpCSCs from both MIAPaCa2 and AsPC1 cells. β- actin used as a loading control.

(B) Western blots analysis demonstrated reduced inhibitory phosphorylation of Gsk3 β at Ser 9 and decreased phosphorylation of Akt at Ser 473 in NpCSCs from both the cell lines. β- actin used as a loading control.

Neu2 modulates Hedgehog (Hh) pathway activity for reduction of stemness property by cross-talking with mTORC2 formation

Formation of mTORC2 is mainly dependent on Rictor. Accordingly, we overexpressed Rictor in the adherent non-stem pancreatic cancer cells and placed them for sphere generation. Rictor overexpression triggered higher and larger spheres formation in both MIAPaCa2 and AsPC1 cells (Fig 5.3A). Next pCSCs were co-expressed with Rictor and Neu2 and we observed less sphere formation (Fig 5.3A). Higher amount of Rictor as well as the mTORC2 formation were observed in Rictor-overexpressed pCSCs compared to pCSCs whereas reduced Rictor and mTORC2 were found in Rictor and Neu2-overexpressed pCSCs (Fig 5.3B). Furthermore, Rictor overexpression in pCSCs resulted to higher expression of pluripotent stem cell markers (Fig 5.4) and Hh-pathway molecules (Fig 5.5), however co-expression of both Rictor and Neu2 reversed these phenomena. Moreover, co-immunoprecipitation of Shh with Patched1 was greatly enhanced upon Rictor overexpression in pCSCs whereas co-expression of both Rictor and Neu2 reduced this association (Fig 5.6). Therefore, Neu2 is capable of directly modulating Hh-pathway as well as mTORC2 formation which are essential characteristics for the survival of pCSCs.

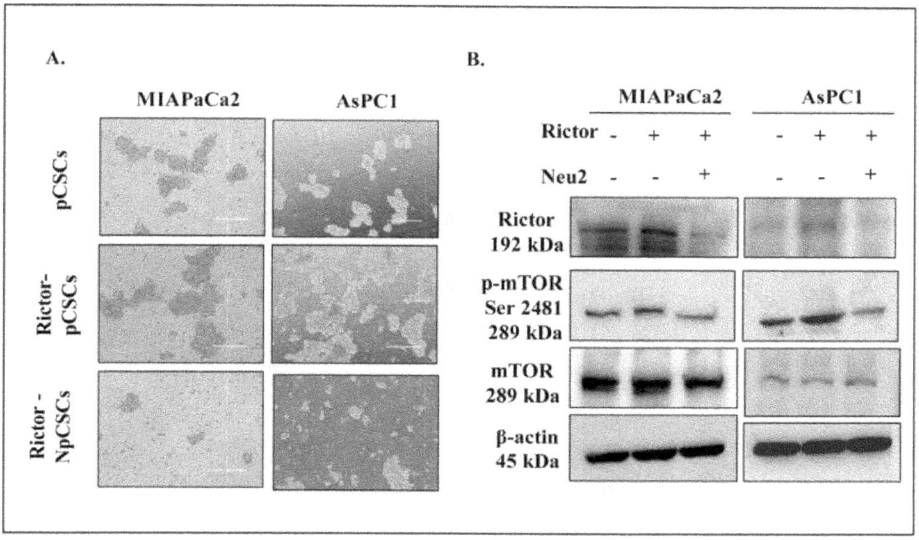

Figure 5.3 (A) Phase contrast images illustrated higher sphere generation upon Rictor overexpression in pCSCs. Co-overexpression of Rictor and Neu2 in pCSCs exhibited reduction of sphere formation.

(B) Representative Immunoblots exhibited enhanced mTORC2 formation and Rictor expression at protein levels in Rictor overexpressed pCSCs whereas reduced expression of these molecules were found in Rictor and Neu2 co-overexpressed pCSCs.

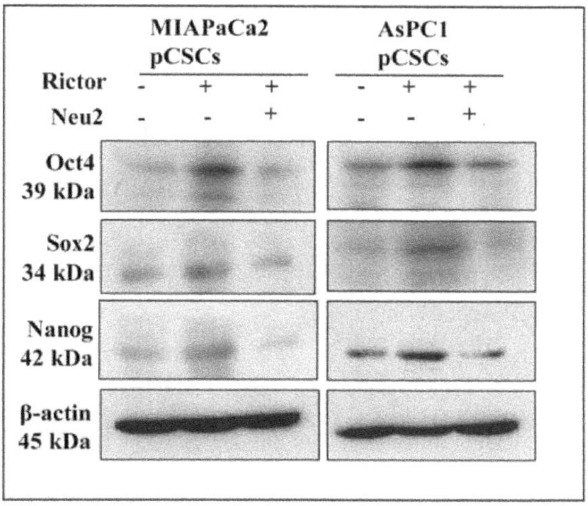

Figure 5.4 Representative Immunoblots showed enhanced expression of Oct4, Sox2 and Nanog at protein level in Rictor overexpressed pCSCs whereas reduced expression of these molecules were observed when both Rictor and Neu2 were co-overexpressed in pCSCs

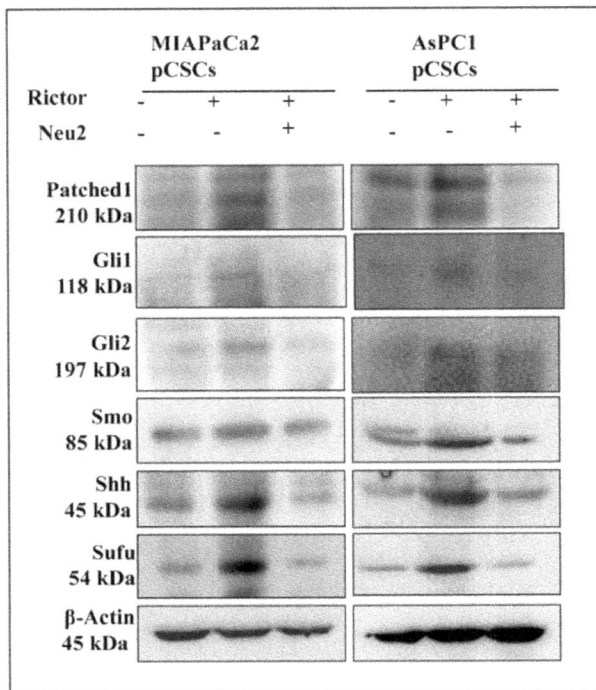

	MIAPaCa2 pCSCs			AsPC1 pCSCs		
Rictor	-	+	+	-	+	+
Neu2	-	-	+	-	-	+

Patched1 210 kDa

Gli1 118 kDa

Gli2 197 kDa

Smo 85 kDa

Shh 45 kDa

Sufu 54 kDa

β-Actin 45 kDa

Figure 5.5 Representative Immunoblots showed increased expression of Hedgehog pathway proteins were observed in Rictor overexpressed pCSCs which were reversed in Rictor and Neu2 co-overexpressed conditions.

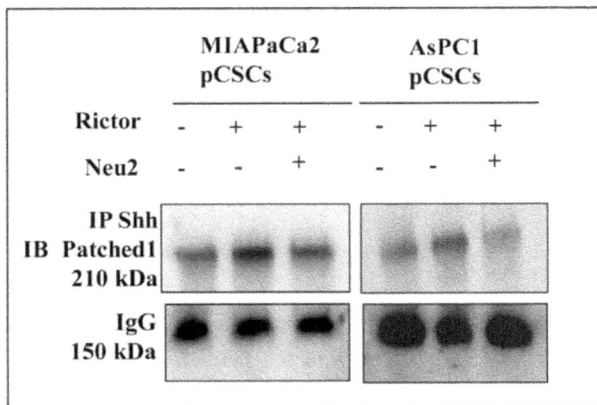

	MIAPaCa2 pCSCs			AsPC1 pCSCs		
Rictor	-	+	+	-	+	+
Neu2	-	-	+	-	-	+

IP Shh IB Patched1 210 kDa

IgG 150 kDa

Figure 5.6 Co-immunoprecipitation of Patched1 and Shh exhibited enhanced association upon Rictor overexpression in pCSCs. Co-overexpression of Rictor and Neu2 in pCSCs exhibited reduction of association of Patched and Shh. Immunoblots of IgG served as loading control.

Neu2-overexpression reduced tumor growth in NOD/SCID mice

For further validation of the effect of Neu2 on apoptosis, we performed *in vivo* tumorigenic experiment in NOD/SCID mice. MIAPaCa2 cells were injected for tumor generation. After formation of tumor, Neu2 plasmid was injected intratumorally for three weeks. Mice were euthanized and tumors were dissected out after 30 days. Neu2-overexpression caused a visible reduction of tumor size in NOD/SCID mice (Fig. 5.7A-B). Results indicated a marked reduction in tumor volume and weight in Neu2-plasmid injected tumors than the vehicle controls (Fig. 5.7C-D). Furthermore, we analyzed the status of a few genes through qPCR analysis of tumor tissues from both vehicle control and Neu2 plasmid injected groups. We observed a significant increase in the mRNA fold change of NEU2 along with a few pro-apoptotic genes such as CASPASE 3/8, and BAX in Neu2-overexpressed tissue samples (Fig. 5.8A). Moreover, Neu2-overexpressed tumor tissue samples showed reduction of pluripotent stem cells markers such as OCT4/SOX2/NANOG and pCSCs specific marker CD133 at genetic level (Fig. 5.8B). Furthermore, we checked the status of Shh and mTOR at protein level. Neu2-overexpressed tumor tissue samples showed a marked decrease of Shh and mTOR at protein level than the vehicle control (Fig. 5.8C). Taken together, Neu2-overexpression into PDAC tumors in NOD/SCID mice led to reduction of tumor growth via modulation of mTOR/Hh axis thereby reducing stemness and induction of apoptosis.

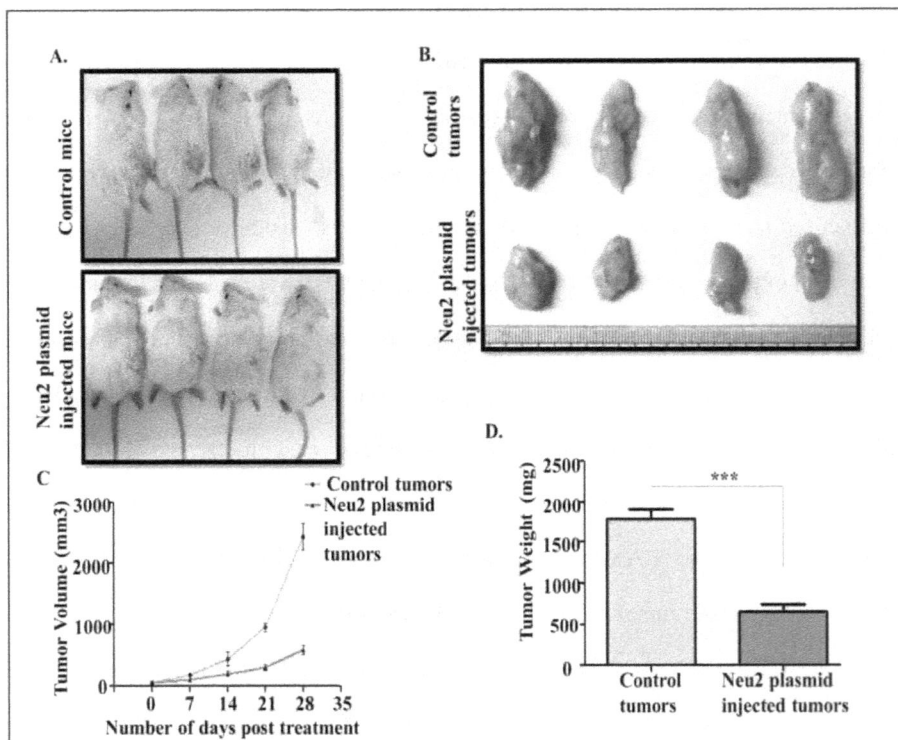

Figure 5.7 (A-D) MIAPaCa-2 (1 X 10[7]) cells were injected subcutaneously into the dorsal side of the right flanks of male NOD/SCID mice to develop tumors. Mice were either injected with vehicle control or 1.5 mg/kg body wt. Neu2-plasmid in admixture with Lipofactamine 2000 (1:2) twice a week for 3 weeks intratumorally. A) Tumor bearing mice, B) Extracted tumors, C) Tumor volume and D) Tumor weights.

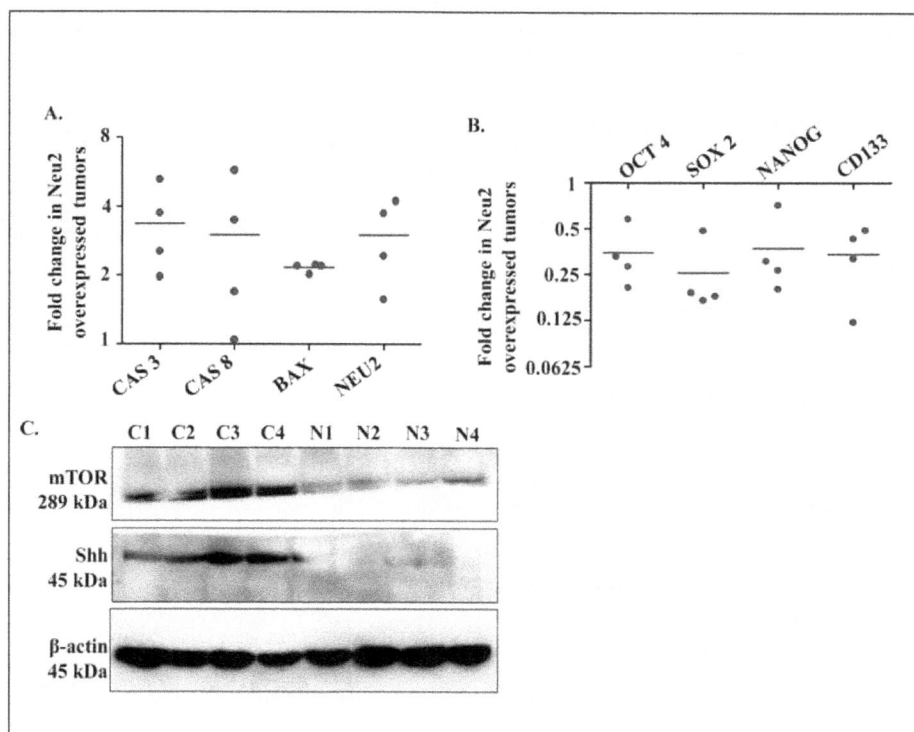

Figure 5.8 (A) Tumor tissues were homogenized and single cells suspension were made and subsequently total RNA was extracted using Trizol. Neu2-overexpression was confirmed at genetic level. qPCR analysis showed up-regulation of pro-apoptotic genes such as CAS 3, CAS 8 and BAX in Neu2-overexpressed tumors.
(B) qPCR data showed down-regulation of pancreatic cancer stem-like cells makers such as OCT4, SOX2, NANOG and CD133 in Neu2-plasmid injected tumor samples.
(C) Tumor tissues were homogenized and whole cells lysates were made. Representative immunoblots illustrated decreased level of Shh and mTOR in Neu2 plasmid injected tumor samples.

5.5 Discussion

We have found reduced mTORC2 formation in Neu2-overexpressed pCSCs and diminished its activity as evidenced by reduced negative phosrylation of GSK3β at Ser 9 position and decreased phosphorylation of AKT at Ser 473 position in NpCSCs. This phenomena also affect the Hh-pathway by ubiquitinylating Gli molecule and ultimately reduced the survival of NpCSCs. Furthermore, Neu2-overexpression in mice tumor tissue also confirmed modulation of stemness properties by Neu2. Overall, our study demonstrate up-regulation of several apoptotic molecules in Neu2-overexpressed pCSCs which conclusively demonstrated the role of sialidase in reduced survival of cancer stem-like cells in pancreatic cancer by modulating both Shh and mTORC2 axis.

We have reported that Neu2 modulates mTORC2 formation in pancreatic cancer cells (chapter III). We had earlier demonstrated a crosstalk between mTORC2 and Hh-pathway in glioblastoma multiforme[47]. Accordingly, in this chapter we have addressed the missing link between mTORC2 and Hh pathway within pCSCs in the context of Neu2-overexpression. We observed higher mTORC2 formation in pCSCs and Neu2-overexpression diminished its activity.

Formation of mTORC2 protein complex is highly dependent on association of Rictor with mTOR[63]. We observed downregulation of Rictor and reduced mTORC2 in NpCSCs. Therefore, crosstalk between Rictor, mTORC2 and Hh pathway in the context of Neu2-overexpression in pancreatic cancer stem-like cells has highlighted their effect in maintaining the stemness property of these cells. Such missing link between mTORC2 and Hh-pathway with respect to the minute balance of sialidases and sialic acids would pave the way for the management of cancer stem-like cells. Here we have observed higher mTORC2 formation and increased Hh activity in pCSCs as demonstrated by enhanced cancer stem cell specific markers in

Rictor-overexpressed condition. To understand the involvement of sialic acids in mTORC2-Hh pathway, we co-expressed both Neu2 and Rictor.

However, even in co-transfected condition, Neu2-overexpression superseded the effect of Rictor-overexpression. Thus, Neu2 plays a dominant role as we have observed reduced mTORC2 as well as several molecules Patched1, Shh, Sufu, Smo, Gli1 and Gli2 in Hh pathway. This clearly demonstrate that overexpressed Neu2 through desialylation of SHH alone or several of these molecules plays significant role in controlling stemness property of NpCSCs as reflected by decreased expression of Oct4, Sox2 and Nanog. Thus we have established a role of Neu2 in mTORC2-Hh pathway axis in NpCSCs. All these events have been demonstrated pictorially in Fig. 5.9.

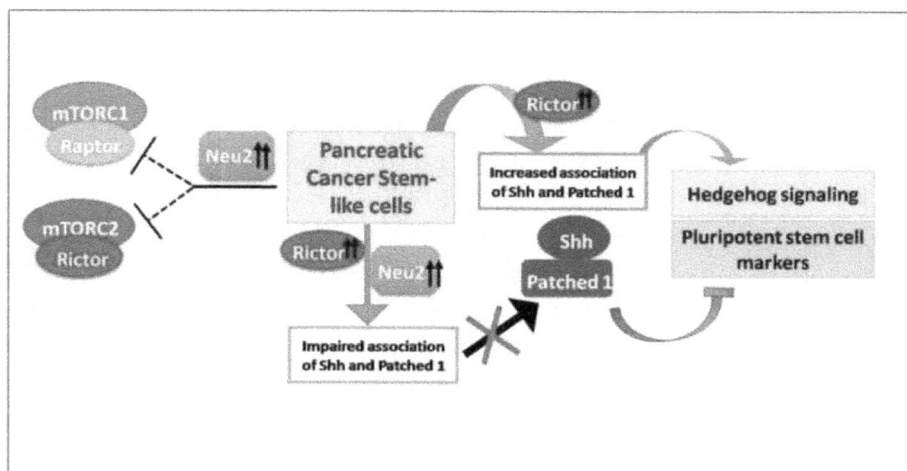

Figure 5.9 Schematic diagram of mechanism of action of Neu2 pCSCs possess higher sialylation and tumorigenic properties than adherent non-stem cancer cells. Overexpression of Neu2 in pCSCs (NpCSCs) leads to a global change in sialylation leading to reduced tumorigenicity. Neu2-overexpression in pCSCs caused desialylation of Shh leading to impaired association with Patched1 thereby reducing Hh signalling and stemness properties. Overexpressed-Neu2 inhibit mTORC1/2 activity thereby inhibit cellular proliferation and subsequently induce apoptosis as corroborated in NOD/SCID mice model.

Furthermore, *in vivo* model in NOD/SCID mice also confirmed modulation of stemness properties and apoptotic molecules by Neu2-overexpression. The data also suggested lower mTOR activity and Shh expression in Neu2 overexpressed tumor tissue sample.

Thus in a nutshell, Neu2-overexpression inhibits the Hh-pathway through Shh desialylation and also by down-regulating mTORC2 formation which helps in activation of GSK3β by down regulating its inhibitory phosphorylation at serine 9 position thus promoting in ubiquitynylation of Gli proteins. Hence, Neu2 is a potential candidate for reducing the stemness of pCSCs.

[This part of the work is currently under review in UGC approved international peer reviewed journal 'MDPI-CELLS']

CHAPTER VI

Conclusion

Pancreatic cancer is a lethal disease because more than 90% patients die due to this cancer, and there are no symptoms during the early stage of this malignant tumor. Although a great amount of effort and research was going on but still the prognosis of this fatal disease is very poor[1]. Currently the ongoing treatments for pancreatic cancer are resection of tumor then followed by chemo and radio therapy, but as this disease is mainly detected in late stage, therefore even after the treatment many patients die. Therefore, significant advance research in the understanding of the molecular pathway could pave the way for the management of this cancer[2].

Abnormal glycosylation, sialylation and fucosylation are very common in cancer which can modulate several biological functions like differentiation, signalling, adhesion, invasiveness, metastasis, and apoptosis [7-11]. Pancreatic cancer exhibits higher sialylation status which affects its elevation in metastasis [13,14]. Enhanced sialic acids mainly depend on the balance of sialic acids modulatory enzymes sialyltransferases and sialidases [15-17]. Modulation of sialylation by sialyltransferases and sialidases plays essential role in carcinogenesis. Till date in mammalian cells four sialidases, which cleave sialic acids from sialylated molecules in cells have been reported, namely lysosomal (Neu1), cytosolic (Neu2), membrane bound (Neu3), and luminal (Neu4) differing in their enzymatic property and substrate specificity[26,27]. These sialidases behave differently during carcinogenesis, however the role of Neu2 remains unexplored in pancreatic-ductal adenocarcinoma (PDAC) and pancreatic cancer stem-like cells (pCSCs). So, we have addressed the effect of Neu2 in PDAC and pCSCS. We have identified low expression of Neu2 is associated with high grade pancreatic ductal adenocarcinoma and a strong-association with clinicopathological-characteristics also its low expression were found in pancreatic cancer stem-like cells. This work aspires us to disclose the modulatory role of sialidase enzyme (Neu2) in controlling different molecular signalling pathways and their cross-talks in pancreatic cancer (PDAC) and pancreatic cancer stem-like cells (pCSCs).

Overexpression of Neu2 induced enhanced apoptosis in PDAC cells (MIAPaCa2 and AsPC1) via extrinsic pathway-mediated apoptotic pathway. This cytosolic sialidase (Neu2) when upregulated it showed its increased enzyme-activity on membrane, and thus it helped in the removal of α2,6-linked sialylation of Fas by direct association. This resulted in activation of Fas, thus resulting in increased apoptosis via activation of FasL, FADD and caspase8.

Up-regulation of PI3K/Akt–mTOR pathway is one of the hallmark pathways of cancer cell survival[37,38]. Neu2-overexpressed PDAC demonstrated inhibition of this pathway probably through by desialylation of some of this pathway molecules, which possibly leads to enhanced Fas expression. Furthermore, Neu2-overexpression caused reduction in cell migration and invasion. So this work connect two signaling hub that interacts with Neu2 one is with Fas mediated extrinsic apoptotic pathway, another is PI3K-Akt-mTOR-signalling hub. This has been summarized in Fig 6.1.

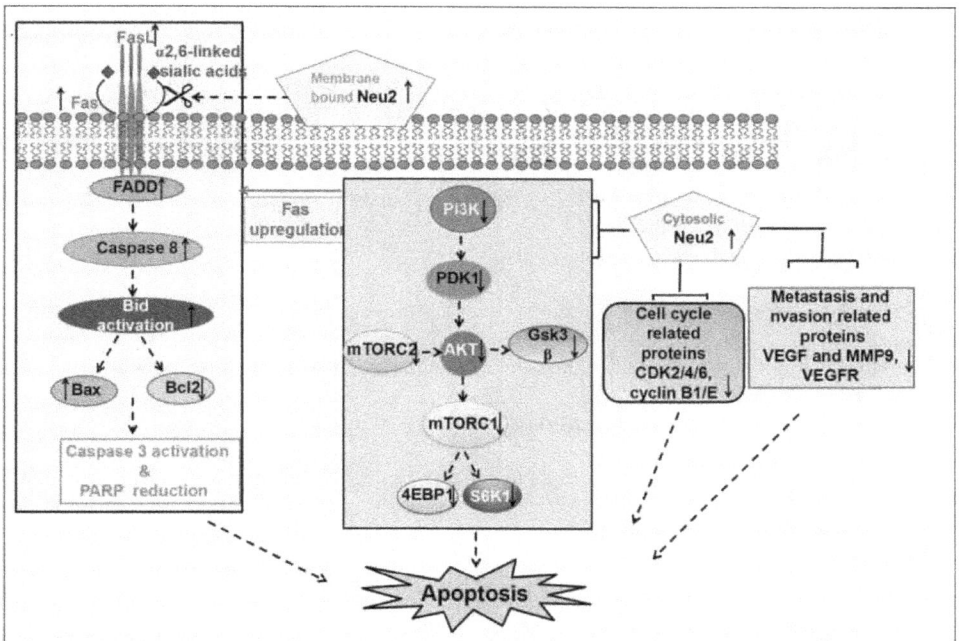

Fig 6.1 Summary of the effect of Neu2-overexpression in pancreatic cancer Cell Death and Disease (2018) 9:210

Revealing of this huge effect on pancreatic cancer apoptosis by Neu2 led us to think whether Neu2 play any specific role for the maintenance of stemness properties of pancreatic cancer stem-like cells (pCSCs). Our research work have revealed that Neu2 up-regulation in pCSCs reduced their stemness properties.

Hedgehog pathway is an important pathway for stem cell survival, relapse and recurrence[43-46]. Neu2-overexpression caused enhanced-association of Neu2 with sonic hedgehog (Shh), which resulted in desialylation of Shh leading to reduced Shh-Patched1 association and decreased expression of hedgehog-pathway. Moreover, for the first time we have reported that Shh is a sialoglycoprotein having $\alpha2,3$-/$\alpha2,6$-linked sialic-acids. These sialic acids on Shh are desialylated by Neu2.

Another major molecule that is associated with cancer progression is mammalian target of rapamycin (mTOR)[61]. The mTOR molecule is known to be upregulated in several cancer which leads to cancer cell proliferation[62]. We have established a close relationship between reduced hedgehog-pathway and decreased mTORC2 formation along with inhibitory-phosphorylation of Gsk3β upon Neu2-overexpression in pCSCs. Lower mTORC2 activity could not inhibit GSK3β from ubiquitination of Gli molecule the major functional molecule of hedgehog pathway resulting in downregulation of this pathway. Moreover, Neu2-overexpression caused reduction in stemness properties in pCSCs by exerting a global effect through modulating Hh-pathway and also via cross-talk between mTORC2 and Hh-pathways. This has been pictorially summarized in Fig 6.2.

Hence, Neu2 may be considered as promising target for the management of pancreatic cancer and pancreatic cancer stem-like cells.

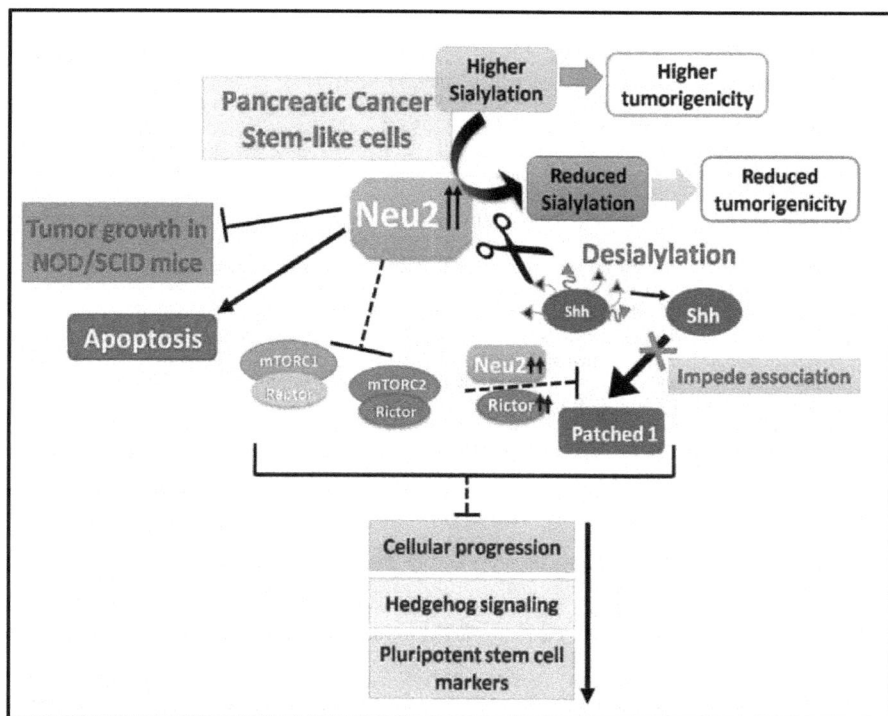

Fig 6.2 Summary of the consequences after Neu2-overexpression in pCSCs.
[This part of the work is currently under review in UGC approved international peer reviewed journal 'MDPI-CELLS']

References:

1. Muders MH, Dutta SK, Wang L, Lau JS, Bhattacharya R, Smyrk TC, et al. Expression and regulatory role of GAIP-interacting protein GIPC in pancreatic adenocarcinoma. Cancer Res 2006; 66: 10264–10268.
2. Muders MH, Vohra PK, Dutta SK, Wang E, Ikeda Y, Wang L, et al. Targeting GIPC/Synectin in Pancreatic Cancer Inhibits Tumor Growth. Clin. Cancer Res. 2009; 15: 4095–4103.
3. Wang Z, Ahmad A, Li Y, Azmi AS, Miele L, Sarkar FH. Targeting notch to eradicate pancreatic cancer stem cells for cancer therapy. Anticancer Res. 2011; 31: 1105–13.
4. Sarkar S, Dutta D, Samanta SK, Bhattacharya K, Pal BC, Li J, et al. Oxidative inhibition of Hsp90 disrupts the super-chaperone complex and attenuates pancreatic adenocarcinoma in vitro and in vivo. Int. J. cancer 2013; 132: 695–706.
5. Sarkar S, Mandal C, Sangwan R, Mandal C. Coupling G2/M arrest to the Wnt/β-catenin pathway restrains pancreatic adenocarcinoma. Endocr. Relat. Cancer 2014; 21: 113–125.
6. Mandal C, Sarkar S, Chatterjee U, Schwartz-Albiez R, Mandal C. Disialoganglioside GD3-synthase over expression inhibits survival and angiogenesis of pancreatic cancer cells through cell cycle arrest at S-phase and disruption of integrin-β1-mediated anchorage. Int. J. Biochem. Cell Biol. 2014; 53: 162–173.
7. Mandal C, Chatterjee M, Sinha D. Investigation of 9-O-acetylated sialoglycoconjugates in childhood acute lymphoblastic leukaemia. Br. J. Haematol. 2000; 110: 801–12.
8. Chowdhury S, Mandal C. O-acetylated sialic acids: multifaceted role in childhood acute lymphoblastic leukaemia. Biotechnol. J. 2009; 4: 361–74.
9. Pal S, Ghosh S, Bandyopadhyay S, Mandal C, Bandhyopadhyay S, Kumar Bhattacharya D, et al. Differential expression of 9-O-acetylated sialoglycoconjugates on leukemic blasts: a potential tool for long-term monitoring of children with acute lymphoblastic leukemia. Int. J. cancer 2004; 111: 270–7.
10. Narayanan S. Sialic acid as a tumor marker. Ann. Clin. Lab. Sci. 1994; 24: 376–84.
11. Büll C, Stoel MA, den Brok MH, Adema GJ. Sialic acids sweeten a tumor's life. Cancer Res. 2014; 74: 3199–3204.
12. Pearce OM, Läubli H. Sialic acids in cancer biology and immunity. Glycobiology 2016; 26: 111–128.
13. Ulloa F, Real FX. Differential distribution of sialic acid in α2, 3 and α2, 6 linkages in the apical membrane of cultured epithelial cells and tissues. J. Histochem. Cytochem. 2001; 49: 501–509.
14. Bassagañas S, Pérez-Garay M, Peracaula R. Cell surface sialic acid modulates extracellular matrix adhesion and migration in pancreatic adenocarcinoma cells. Pancreas 2014; 43: 109–17.
15. Monti E, Bonten E, D'Azzo A, Bresciani R, Venerando B, Borsani G, et al. Sialidases in Vertebrates. A Family Of Enzymes Tailored For Several Cell Functions. Advances in Carbohydrate Chemistry and Biochemistry 2010; 64: 403-79.
16. Mandal, C. Regulation of O-acetylation of sialic acids by sialate-O-acetyltransferase and sialate-O-acetylesterase activities in childhood acute lymphoblastic leukemia. Glycobiology 2012; 22: 70–83.
17. Mondal S, Chandra S, Mandal C. Elevated mRNA level of hST6Gal I and hST3Gal V positively correlates with the high risk of pediatric acute leukemia. Leuk. Res. 2010; 34: 463–470.
18. Mandal C, Srinivasan GV, Chowdhury S, Chandra S, Mandal C, Schauer R, et al. High level of sialate-O-acetyltransferase activity in lymphoblasts of childhood acute lymphoblastic leukaemia (ALL): enzyme characterization and correlation with disease status. Glycoconj. J. 2009; 26: 57–73.
19. Glavey SV, Manier S, Natoni A, Sacco A, Moschetta M, Reagan MR, et al. The sialyltransferase ST3GAL6 influences homing and survival in multiple myeloma. Blood 2014; 124: 1765–1776.
20. Harvey BE, Toth CA, Wagner HE, Steele GD Jr, Thomas P.Sialyltransferase activity and hepatic tumor growth in a nude mouse model of colorectal cancer metastases. Cancer Res 1992; 52: 1775–1779.
21. Zhao Y, Wei A, Zhang H, Chen X, Wang L, Zhang H, et al. α2,6-Sialylation mediates hepatocellular carcinoma growth in vitro and in vivo by targeting the Wnt/β-catenin pathway. Oncogenesis 2017; 6: e343.
22. Cao Y, Merling A, Crocker PR, Keller R, Schwartz-Albiez R.Differential expression of beta-galactoside alpha2,6 sialyltransferase and sialoglycans in normal and cirrhotic liver and hepatocellular carcinoma. Lab. Invest. 2002; 82: 1515–1524.
23. Bassagañas S, Carvalho S, Dias AM, Pérez-Garay M, Ortiz MR, Figueras J, et al. Pancreatic cancer cell glycosylation regulates cell adhesion and invasion through the modulation of α2β1 integrin and E-cadherin function. PLoS One 2014; 9: (5): e98595.
24. Chi-Che Hsieh, Yi-Ming Shyr, Wen-Ying Liao, Tien-Hua Chen, Shin-E Wang, Peir-Chuen Lu, et al. Elevation of β-galactoside α2 , 6-sialyltransferase 1 in a fructose- responsive manner promotes pancreatic cancer metastasis. Oncotarget 2016; 8: 7691–7709.
25. Pérez-Garay M, Arteta B, Llop E, Cobler L, Pagès L, Ortiz R, et al. α2,3-Sialyltransferase ST3Gal IV promotes migration and metastasis in pancreatic adenocarcinoma cells and tends to be highly expressed in pancreatic adenocarcinoma tissues. Int. J. Biochem. Cell Biol. 2013; 45: 1748–1757.
26. Miyagi T. Aberrant expression of sialidase and cancer progression. Proc. Jpn. Acad. Ser. B. Phys. Biol. Sci. 2008; 84: 407–18.

27. Mandal C, Tringali C, Mondal S, Anastasia L, Chandra S, Venerando B, et al. Down regulation of membrane-bound Neu3 constitutes a new potential marker for childhood acute lymphoblastic leukemia and induces apoptosis suppression of neoplastic cells. Int. J. cancer 2010; 126: 337–49.

28. Koseki K, Wada T, Hosono M, Hata K, Yamaguchi K, Nitta K, et al. Human cytosolic sialidase NEU2-low general tissue expression but involvement in PC-3 prostate cancer cell survival. Biochem. Biophys. Res. Commun. 2012; 428: 142–9.

29. Fanzani A, Colombo F, Giuliani R, Preti A, Marchesini S. Cytosolic sialidase Neu2 upregulation during PC12 cells differentiation. FEBS Lett. 2004; 566: 178–182.

30. Fanzani A, Giuliani R, Colombo F, Zizioli D, Presta M, Preti A, et al. Overexpression of cytosolic sialidase Neu2 induces myoblast differentiation in C2C12 cells. FEBS Lett. 2003; 547: 183–188.

31. Von Reyher U, Sträter J, Kittstein W, Gschwendt M, Krammer PH, Möller P. Colon carcinoma cells use different mechanisms to escape CD95-mediated apoptosis. Cancer Res 1998; 58: 526–534.

32. Keane MM1, Ettenberg SA, Lowrey GA, Russell EK, Lipkowitz S. Fas expression and function in normal and malignant breast cell lines. Cancer Res. 1996; 56: 4791–4798.

33. Swindall A. F,Bellis, S. L. Sialylation of the Fas Death Receptor by ST6Gal-I Provides Protection against Fas-mediated Apoptosis in Colon Carcinoma Cells. J. Biol. Chem. 2011; 286: 22982–22990.

34. Sadeghi N, GerberD. E. Targeting the PI3K pathway for cancer therapy. Future Med. Chem. 2012; 4: 1153–1169.

35. MorgenszternD, McLeod, H. L. PI3K/Akt/mTOR pathway as a target for cancer therapy. Anticancer. Drugs 2005; 16: 797–803.

36. Zhao Y, Li Y, Ma H, Dong W, Zhou H, Song X, et al. Modification of sialylation mediates the invasive properties and chemosensitivity of human hepatocellular carcinoma. Mol. Cell. Proteomics 2014; 13: 520–36.

37. Ma H, Zhou H, Song X, Shi S, Zhang J, Jia L. Modification of sialylation is associated with multidrug resistance in human acute myeloid leukemia. Oncogene 2014; 34: 1–15.

38. Osaki M, Kase S, Adachi K, Takeda A, Hashimoto K, Ito H. Inhibition of the PI3K-Akt signaling pathway enhances the sensitivity of Fas-mediated apoptosis in human gastric carcinoma cell line, MKN-45. J. Cancer Res. Clin. Oncol. 2004; 130: 8–14.

39. Zhu L, Derijard B, Chakrabandhu K, Wang BS, Chen HZ, Hueber AO. Synergism of PI3K/Akt inhibition and Fas activation on colon cancer cell death. Cancer Lett. 2014; 354: 355–364.

40. Bertram J, Peacock JW, Tan C, Mui AL, Chung SW, Gleave ME, et al. Inhibition of the phosphatidylinositol 3'-kinase pathway promotes autocrine Fas-induced death of phosphatase and tensin homologue-deficient prostate cancer cells. Cancer Res. 2006; 66: 4781–4788.

41. Tringali C, Lupo B, Anastasia L, Papini N, Monti E, Bresciani R, et al. Expression of sialidase Neu2 in leukemic K562 cells induces apoptosis by impairing Bcr-Abl/Src kinases signaling. J. Biol. Chem. 2007; 282: 14364–14372.

42. Miyagi T, Takahashi K, Hata K, Shiozaki K. Yamaguchi K. Sialidase significance for cancer progression. Glycoconj. J. 2012; 29: 567–577.

43. Mondal S, Bhattacharya K, Mandal C. Nutritional stress reprograms dedifferention in glioblastoma multiforme driven by PTEN/Wnt/Hedgehog axis: a stochastic model of cancer stem cells. Cell Death Discov. 2018; 4:110.

44. Plaks V, Kong N, Werb Z. The cancer stem cell niche: how essential is the niche in regulating stemness of tumor cells? Cell Stem Cell. 2015; 16(3):225-38.

45. Tang SN, Fu J, Nall D, Rodova M, Shankar S, Srivastava RK. Inhibition of sonic hedgehog pathway and pluripotency maintaining factors regulate human pancreatic cancer stem cell characteristics. Int J Cancer. 2012;131(1):30–40.

46. Merchant AA, Matsui W. Targeting Hedgehog--a cancer stem cell pathway. Clin Cancer Res. 2010;16(12):3130–3140.

47. Maiti S, Mondal S, Satyavarapu EM, Mandal C. mTORC2 regulates hedgehog pathway activity by promoting stability to Gli2 protein and its nuclear translocation. Cell Death Dis. 2017;8(7):e2926.

48. Miyazaki Y, Matsubara S, Ding Q, Tsukasa K, Yoshimitsu M, Kosai K, et al. Efficient elimination of pancreatic cancer stem cells by hedgehog/GLI inhibitor GANT61 in combination with mTOR inhibition. Mol Cancer. 2016; 15(1):49.

49. Zuo M, Rashid A, Churi C, Vauthey JN, Chang P, Li Y, et al. Novel therapeutic strategy targeting the Hedgehog signalling and mTOR pathways in biliary tract cancer. Br J Cancer. 2015; 112(6):1042-51.

50. Skoda AM, Simovic D, Karin V, Kardum V, Vranic S, Serman L. The role of the Hedgehog signaling pathway in cancer: A comprehensive review. Bosn J Basic Med Sci. 2018;18(1):8-20.

51. Aponte PM, Caicedo A. Stemness in Cancer: Stem Cells, Cancer Stem Cells, and Their Microenvironment. Stem Cells Int. 2017; 2017:5619472.

52. Lathia JD, Liu H. Overview of Cancer Stem Cells and Stemness for Community Oncologists. Target Oncol. 2017 Aug;12(4):387-399.

53. Nath S, Mandal C, Chatterjee U, Mandal C. Association of cytosolic sialidase Neu2 with plasma membrane enhances Fas-mediated apoptosis by impairing PI3K-Akt/mTOR-mediated pathway in pancreatic cancer cells. Cell Death Dis. 2018; 9(2):210.
54. Razi E, Radak M, Mahjoubin Tehran M, Talebi S, Shafiee A, Hajighadimi S, et al. Cancer stem cells as therapeutic targets of pancreatic cancer. Fundam Clin Pharmacol. 2019.
55. Barkeer S, Chugh S, Batra SK, Ponnusamy MP. Glycosylation of Cancer Stem Cells: Function in Stemness, Tumorigenesis, and Metastasis. Neoplasia. 2018; 20(8):813-825.
56. Schultz MJ, Holdbrooks AT, Chakraborty A, Grizzle WE, Landen CN, Buchsbaum DJ, et al. The Tumor-Associated Glycosyltransferase ST6Gal-I Regulates Stem Cell Transcription Factors and Confers a Cancer Stem Cell Phenotype. Cancer Res. 2016; 76(13):3978-88.
57. Wang YC, Stein JW, Lynch CL, Tran HT, Lee CY, Coleman R, et al. Glycosyltransferase ST6GAL1 contributes to the regulation of pluripotency in human pluripotent stem cells. Sci Rep. 2015; 5:13317.
58. Wang F, Ma L, Zhang Z, Liu X, Gao H, Zhuang Y, et al. Hedgehog Signalling Regulates Epithelial-Mesenchymal Transition in Pancreatic Cancer Stem-Like Cells. J Cancer. 2016;7(4):408-17.
59. Li C, Du Y, Yang Z, He L, Wang Y, Hao L et al. GALNT1-Mediated Glycosylation and Activation of Sonic Hedgehog Signalling Maintains the Self-Renewal and Tumor-Initiating Capacity of Bladder Cancer Stem Cells. Cancer Res. 2016; 76(5):1273-83.
60. Carballo GB, Honorato JR, de Lopes GPF, Spohr TCLSE. A highlight on Sonic hedgehog pathway. Cell Commun Signal. 2018;16(1):11.
61. Francipane MG, Lagasse E. Therapeutic potential of mTOR inhibitors for targeting cancer stem cells. Br J Clin Pharmacol. 2016 Nov;82(5):1180-1188.
62. Matsubara S, Ding Q, Miyazaki Y, Kuwahata T, Tsukasa K, Takao S. mTOR plays critical roles in pancreatic cancer stem cells through specific and stemness-related functions. Sci Rep. 2013 Nov 15;3:3230.
63. Bhattacharya K, Maiti S, Mandal C. PTEN negatively regulates mTORC2 formation and signalling in grade IV glioma via Rictor hyperphosphorylation at Thr1135 and direct the mode of action of an mTORC1/2 inhibitor. Oncogenesis. 2016; 5(5):e227.

www.ingramcontent.com/pod-product-compliance
Lightning Source LLC
Chambersburg PA
CBHW070521030426

42337CB00016B/2051